MEDITERRANEAN DIET FOR BEGINNERS 1:

62 Breakfast & lunch recipes.

The most delicious and traditional way to start
dieting. Enjoy amazing dishes while losing weight.
(with 31 bonus meal plans included)

Lily Attridge

INTRODUCTION

Healthy living is a treasured luxury that doesn't come by itself. You have to schedule it. Nutrition plays a crucial role in supplying the body with essential nutrients for growth and development. While some foods are considered healthy and in large quantities are required, others may be excluded from a daily diet. So works a Mediterranean diet plan.

The most common type of healthy diet is the Mediterranean diet. Studies have proven that people in the Mediterranean region can attribute the secret of healthy living to their balanced diet and active lifestyles. Researches have also shown that not only does this diet alleviate chronic heart disease, it also increases life expectancy.

Today's habits show that most people prefer to eat fried, frozen, or tinned foods that contain saturated fats and sugar. Lifestyles often suggest that most people don't take the time to exercise. As a result, with an increased chance of heart disease, diabetes, and cancers, many people are obese and unhealthy.

The Mediterranean diet plan does not reduce the food types that one eats. The diet advises wise choices regarding food. For starters, instead of tinned and frozen food, one should eat fresh fruit and vegetables.

The food plan is based on the pyramid Mediterranean diet. According to him, cereals, grains, pasta, vegetables, legumes, beans, fruit, and nuts are food products to be included in a daily diet. These nutritious goods are a rich source of carbohydrates, fabrics, vitamins, minerals, and proteins. The recommended milk, yogurt, and cheese consumption, low to moderate, reduce excessive intake of saturated fats. Animal meat such as chicken and eggs shall be consumed regularly and red meat, several times a month. Fish is considered a better choice since it is high in nutritional value.

Olive oil provides good fat, which is responsible for reducing blood cholesterol levels and maintaining a healthy heart. All these recommendations are in line with a regular diet recommendation in the Mediterranean diet plan. A balanced dietary intake through an active physical life. This is not to say that people did not find time to rest in the Mediterranean area. They also used the time to relax and socialize after each meal, unwittingly giving time for proper digestion and good health.

CHAPTER 1

INTRODUCTION TO MEDITERRANEAN DIET

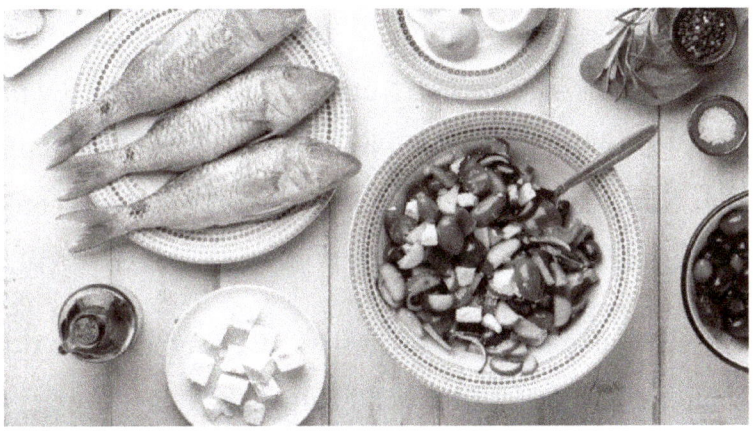

The Mediterranean diet is more than a diet. It is a lifestyle. It's a way of eating to live a full and healthy life. When following this way of eating you'll not only lose weight, but you'll also strengthen your heart and provide your body with all the proper nutrients necessary to live a long and productive life. People following the Mediterranean diet have been linked to a lower risk of Alzheimer's disease and cancer, better overall cardiovascular health, and an extended lifespan. The building blocks that comprise a Mediterranean diet are foods rich in healthy oils, low in saturated fat, and filled with vegetables and fresh fruits.

The Mediterranean diet focuses on typical foods and recipes you'd find in Mediterranean-style cooking. Here's what goes into the Mediterranean diet. This diet includes consuming lots of vegetables and grains, fruits, rice, and pasta while limiting fats, replacing salt with herbs and spices, and eating fish and poultry instead of red meat. The Mediterranean diet does not contain a lot of red meat. Nuts are a part of a healthy part of this diet. However, one should limit themselves to a handful or so a day. Nuts have a high amount of fat, but a high percentage of fat isn't saturated.

Nuts are also high in calories so carefully monitor the amount you eat. You'll want to avoid salted nuts and honey roasted or candied nuts.

It may even include a glass of red wine per day, and regular physical activities to fully maximize the remarkable health benefits. The Mediterranean diet reflects various eating habits of the countries near the Mediterranean Sea, mainly Southern Italy, Greece, Morocco, France, and Spain. Due to their unique locality, the climate supports fresh fruits, vegetables, and some of the world's best seafood.

This diet isn't focused on limiting your total consumption of fat, instead, it focuses on making smarter choices about the kinds of fat you consume. This diet discourages people from eating trans-fats and saturated fats, both of which have been linked to heart disease.

Grains used in the Mediterranean diet are preferably whole grain, which generally contains very little in the way of unhealthy trans-fat. Bread is an important part of the Mediterranean lifestyle; however, bread should not be covered in margarine or butter. Instead, the bread is eaten either dipped in olive oil or eaten plain. This cuts down significantly on some trans and saturated fats normally associated with eating bread.

Wine plays a large role in the Mediterranean diet. A glass of wine is normally included with each evening meal.

This means 5 ounces or less of wine for anyone over the age of 65 and for people under 65 no more than 10 ounces daily. If you have any history of alcohol dependency or abuse, I suggest refraining altogether from consuming alcohol as part of your diet. The same goes if you already have liver or heart disease.

Olive oil is the primary source of fat in this type of diet. It provides monounsaturated fat, which is the kind of fat that helps reduce the levels of LDL cholesterol when utilized instead of trans or saturated fats. The "Extra virgin" and "virgin" olive oils are considered to have undergone the least processing. They also happen to contain the largest levels of protective plant compounds responsible for providing antioxidant effects.

What is LDL?

Cholesterol is a compound belonging to the sterol or steroid alcohol subgroup of organic molecules. It is classified as a waxy steroid of fat. It is an essential component of cellular membranes and a precursor to the production of fat-soluble vitamins, such as vitamin D.

There are two main types of cholesterol; HDL (high-density lipoproteins) and LDL (low-density lipoproteins). Though this is not entirely accurate. HDL and LDL are lipoproteins. They are the transport mechanisms for cholesterol particles. They are composed of proteins and fats.

LDL particles transport cholesterols from the liver to the cells of the body.

HDLs collect any that are found in the tissues or produced by other organs and carry it back to the liver for reprocessing.

This is why HDLs are sometimes referred to as "good" cholesterol because they pick up any that are dropped in the bloodstream before it can adhere to the walls of the arteries. LDL is known as bad cholesterol.

Although it is essential for life, large amounts of cholesterol in the bloodstream may increase a person's risk of heart disease, mainly atherosclerosis. This is why balance in HDL/LDL particles is so important, and an imbalance can be dangerous.

Highlight on Trans-fats

Trans-fats are listed as hydrogenated or partially hydrogenated oils. The oils may be soy, canola or simply listed as partially hydrogenated "vegetable" il. This kind of fat is the worst kind you can eat.

According to the Mayo Clinic, trans-fats raise LDL levels and lowers HDL levels. It is a man-made fat that is found in baked goods and other packaged foods. In addition to causing HDL/LDL imbalance, it raises total blood triglycerides (fats that normally circulate in the bloodstream) and promotes plaque buildup on arterial walls. Like obesity, trans-fat also contributes to chronic inflammation.

Another major component of the Mediterranean diet is fatty fish.

This includes lake trout, salmon, sardines, herring, mackerel, and albacore tuna. They have plenty of omega-3 fatty acids.

This type of fatty acid helps to decrease blood clotting and lower our triglyceride levels. High triglyceride levels (more than 150 mg/dL) can cause heart diseases. Omega-3 fatty acids are also associated with helping to moderate blood pressure, decrease the risk of sudden heart attack, and improve the overall health of our blood vessels.

I often get asked how many times per week can eat certain types of foods. Well, on the Mediterranean diet you can enjoy foods like yogurt, cheese, vegetables, whole grains, beans, and fruits daily. However, fish, eggs, and meat should only be served once or twice each week. You'll find that this is easier to do than you think, especially after a couple of weeks once you've readjusted to your new way of eating. I have a ton of delicious recipes you can try out in later chapters.

The Mediterranean diet is 35 to 40 percent fat. However, the diet is focused primarily on healthy fats. Though higher in calories, fats make your food taste better and your meals feel more satisfying. You will eat a little less but enjoy your food significantly more.

I often hear people ask if they'll always feel hungry when following this diet. The answer to that is a resounding "NO."

Since the Mediterranean diet places emphasis on high fiber nutrients rich foods like vegetables, beans, fresh fruits, legumes, and whole grains you'll never have the intense hunger pangs associated with so many other diets on the market. You may be eating less each day, but your stomach won't feel that way.

The Mediterranean lifestyle itself plays a large role in

supporting your diet plan. You'll want to get plenty of exercise but still carve out time to have long leisurely meals with your family and friends.

The good thing about the Mediterranean diet is that it doesn't require you to buy any special kind of food. No money will be wasted on buying foods that are labeled as being low-fat or diet. Though there are exceptions, a Mediterranean diet consists of less processed, natural food. The more natural foods you incorporate into your daily diet, the healthier you'll be.

Being on a Mediterranean diet requires commitment. You'll be spending more time preparing your meals in your kitchen. Since you're eating natural foods, they won't already be processed and ready to go. I suggest brushing up on your cooking skills or taking a class if you have no skills to speak of. I love to cook so this wasn't too big of a change for me. However, I have friends who had zero skills in the kitchen, and they found this to be a daunting challenge at first.

I plan out my weekly meals on Friday nights. Each Saturday I shop for all my food and then I prepare the majority of my meals in advance on Sunday.

Having a schedule and system in place makes the entire process go much smoother. It also ensures I always have a healthy meal on hand in case I'm feeling unmotivated to cook for myself at certain times of the week.

As with most diets, it's also very important to stay well hydrated when on this diet. Drink 64 oz. or 8 glasses of water daily. If you ever feel like you're getting a headache or a muscle cramp, you may just need some water.

I also suggest keeping a daily log of your meals. I go over what I use in the resources section. Keeping track of what you're eating is a good tool to help keep you motivated and on point. It will be a good way to identify the things throw you off course. For instance, when I first started, I noticed my food intake was terrible on Sunday.

This was because for much of the year I would spend Sunday afternoons watching football with friends while eating and drinking non-stop. Once I saw what I was consuming compared to the rest of my week, I knew what changes I needed to make to keep me on track.

Don't forget to check with your physician before starting this diet. I know it sounds like a giant hassle, but you should always determine a proper course of action with a trained professional before getting started.

Major Features of a Mediterranean Diet:

- The primary source of your fat in this diet is olive oil.

- Dinner often includes a glass of red wine.

- Vegetables and seasonal fresh fruits are a major part of every meal.

- Whole grain pasta and bread are served without any type of apology,

- Meat is consumed in smaller portions, and red meat is primarily avoided altogether.

- Popular flavors include garlic, basil, oregano, lemon, rosemary, and mint.

CHAPTER 2

ADVANTAGES AND DISADVANTAGES OF MEDITERRANEAN DIET

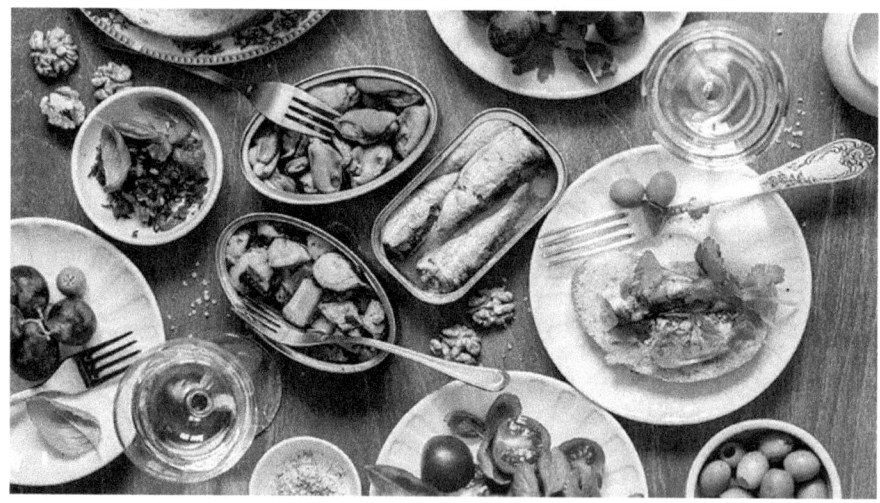

Benefits Of The Mediterranean Diet

Many studies prove the many advantages of the Mediterranean Diet. However, even if you don't look at the studies, the Mediterranean people serve as first-hand proof of the benefits of this wonderful diet. Here are many benefits of going on the Mediterranean Diet.

Long and Healthy Life

The Mediterranean cuisine is often referred to as the healthiest cuisine in the world, and the diet doesn't stray too far away. Being based mostly on fresh vegetables and fruits, healthy oils and whole grains, as well as lean meat and seafood, it's not hard to see why this diet is considered to be healthy. Mix with a glass of red wine, and you've got yourself a fun, easy-going diet.

Your Heart Will Thank You

Scientific evidence easily connects good heart health with certain foods, mainly vegetables, fruits, olive oil, and nuts. The Mediterranean diet has it all!

The Mediterranean diet is all about highlighting healthy fats. Instead of using the usual cooking oil, the diet uses olive oil which contains healthy fat that is good for the heart. With that said, the Mediterranean Diet can help decrease your risk of heart failure.

A Mediterranean diet consists of food with monounsaturated fats like olive oil rather than saturated fats like butter.

The Mediterranean diet naturally includes most of the key diet changes that would keep your heart in tip-top shape

Shed Some Unwanted Weight

Although the main focus of this diet is not weight loss, it will surely help with it if that's what you're looking for. Just look at it from this point of view: fresh, clean food combined with whole grains, good fats, less sugar and plenty of liquids coupled with copious amounts of exercise. By transitioning to healthy foods and a healthy lifestyle, you'll shed pounds without causing drastic imbalances in your body. Also, it is known that plant-based diets like the Mediterranean diet are really helpful in losing weight. The mere fact that you stopped eating junk food and processed food with sugar and unhealthy fats is already a very good start to weight loss!

Controls Diabetes

Because it focuses on fresh ingredients and it packs plenty of vitamins, antioxidants, and minerals, this diet is a great way to keep your diabetes under control. This lifestyle controls excess insulin, which in turn lowers our blood sugar levels.

Regulating blood sugar levels is vastly important to living a healthier lifestyle.

There is a need for balancing a lot of whole foods into this plan to find quality sources of protein and consume carbs that are low in sugar. That makes the body burn fat much more efficiently, and you will have more energy as a result.

In short, a natural diet with fresh produce is a natural combater of diabetes.

It is Affordable

The Mediterranean diet is accessible even if you're on a budget. Legumes, vegetables, fruits, herbs, whole grains, and olive oil are not as expensive as they sound, but they offer so much versatility in the kitchen.

Boost Brain Power

The Mediterranean Diet can also counteract the brain's poor ability to perform. Choosing this lifestyle will help you preserve your memory, leading to an overall increase in your cognitive health.

Normally cognitive disorders are caused by a scenario where your brain is unable to get a sufficient amount of dopamine.

Dopamine is a compound or chemical present in the brain responsible for passing information from one neuron to the other. It is responsible for thought processing, mood regulation, and proper body movements.

The ability of the Mediterranean diet to help boost your cognitive health is normally linked to the combination of its anti-inflammatory fruits and vegetables, its healthy fats and nuts.

These foods normally battle cognitive decline that is caused by age. But how do these foods do it?

These foods normally deal with elements that cause impaired brain function like inflammation, free radicals, and exposure to toxicity.

Fatty fish, nuts and olive oils all contain omega 3 fatty acids that usually help reduce the level of inflammation in your body. Such vegetables like spinach, kale, and broccoli that are dark green contain vitamin E, which is known to protect your body from an anti-inflammatory molecule known as cytokines.

Vegetables like spinach, broccoli, and fruits like raspberries, cherries, and watermelon all have antioxidants that neutralize free radicals that affect your brain. The Mediterranean diet also tends to focus on monounsaturated fats which come from oils like olive oil. The oils and the fatty acids that you get from omega 3 (from fish) combine to keep your arteries unblocked.

That automatically increases the health of your brain and reduces your risk of getting diseases like Alzheimer's disease and dementia.

Encourage Relaxation

The Mediterranean Diet surprisingly enough can encourage relaxation. The diet can lower your levels of insulin and make you feel at ease. High blood sugar can cause you to be hyperactive and later crash; but eating balanced meals with lots of whole grains, fruits, veggies, etc. helps stabilize blood sugar, allowing you to relax and rest. Since a major component of this lifestyle is eating with the family at the dinner table, relaxation is maximized. With a home-cooked meal in your comfort zone, relaxation will be evident with this diet.

Enhance Your Mood

The diet can help you to be positive, even when things aren't going your way. Healthy living does that. When you have eaten enough food to fuel you with lots of nutrients, your body notices. Fulfillment and productivity enhance your mood. For one, applying the diet correctly will make you feel like you're doing something good for yourself, and thus enhances your overall mood.

Improve Skin Condition

Fish have Omega-3 fatty acids. They strengthen the skin membrane and make it more elastic and firmer. Olive oil, red wine, and tomatoes contain a lot of antioxidants to protect against skin damage brought about by chemical reactions and prolonged sun exposure.

Disadvantages Of The Mediterranean Diet:

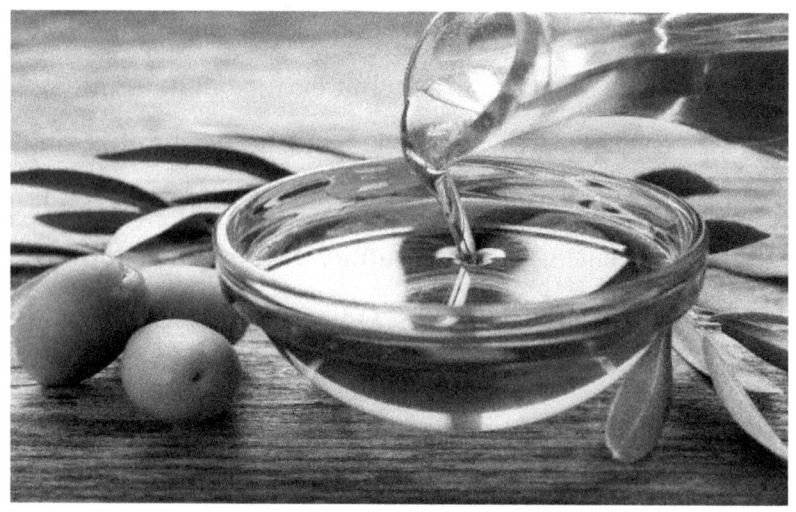

While the Mediterranean Diet has incredible benefits and has proven to be effective in keeping terminal illnesses at bay for generations, it's worth noting that it also has some disadvantages. After all, a perfect diet does not exist.

Not Specific. The Mediterranean works its magic and all, but it's the spell you need to know to make it work. However, the diet does not have a specific "spell." For instance, the foods in the diet vary as the different Mediterranean countries and cities use different varieties of it. For example, Greece and Italy have different preferred food on their tables. There are no official and exact names of certain foods to eat; it only shows generic terminology like fruits, vegetables, fish, and more. Additionally, it doesn't show how much to eat so it could get quite tricky to know exactly if you've overeaten or if you did not follow the diet at all.

Not for some people. Some of the foods included in the diet have gluten, and some people are sensitive to gluten. People with peanut and seafood allergies would also find it hard to follow the Mediterranean Diet as nuts and fish are a major part of the diet. Also, as the diet could require planning the menu and preparing the dishes at home, those who don't have time to cook will find it challenging to follow this.

Not an overnighter. The Mediterranean people are as healthy as they are because their diet is traditional; they have been on it their whole lives. So if you expect results after one day, reign in those unrealistic expectations. In order to get positive, long-lasting results, don't let the Mediterranean Diet be just a passing diet craze. You have to breathe it, live it, and eat it; just like real Mediterranean people.

CHAPTER 3

INGREDIENTS AND NUTRITIONAL VALUES

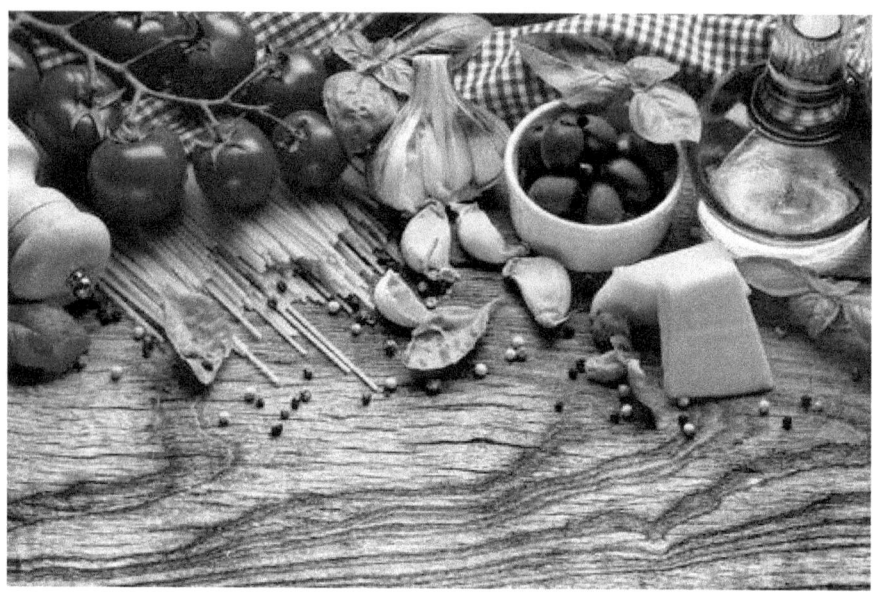

The Mediterranean Diet food pyramid was created 25 years ago by Oldways, a nonprofit food and nutrition education organization. This visual shows which foods are recommended daily and how many servings of each to eat.

FOODS TO FOCUS ON

Vegetables and fruits: Plant foods make up the bulk of the diet and form the largest part of the pyramid. Plants contain special components called phytonutrients that ward off diseases and insects. When we eat the plants, those phytonutrients can help us ward off diseases as well. Fiber-rich fruits and veggies can decrease the risk of chronic diseases and bulk up our meals so we feel full and satisfied.

Nuts and seeds: While nuts and seeds contain some protein, they are mainly composed of monounsaturated and polyunsaturated fats—the healthy fats that can decrease disease risk. Whole nuts and seeds also contain fiber, protein, and phytonutrients.

Beans, legumes, and whole grains: Lentils, cannellini beans, pinto beans, black beans, and chickpeas (garbanzo beans) are used often in Mediterranean meals. They are rich in protein, fiber, and energy-producing B vitamins. Eating more beans and legumes, along with whole grains, is associated with lower disease risk.

Olives and olive oil: Following the Mediterranean Diet means eating olives and/or olive oil daily. Olives are rich in heart-healthy monounsaturated fatty acids and antioxidants. Additionally, the olive fruit (yes, it's a fruit) contains healthy amounts of fiber and iron.

Herbs and spices: Along with providing powerful phytonutrients, many herbs and spices contribute to the unique flavor profiles found in Mediterranean cooking. Using a variety of herbs and spices will increase the nutrition, color, and fresh flavors in your meals.

Oily fish and seafood: There's a reason that seafood gets an important spot on the Mediterranean Diet pyramid: eating seafood two to three times per week reduces the risk of death from any health-related cause, according to a 2006 study in the Journal of the American Medical Association. It's essential during pregnancy and helps children develop a healthy brain and eyes, as outlined in a 2007 study in The Lancet. It's also linked to improved memory in older adults, according to a 2012 study in Neurology. The essential omega-3 fats in fish are found in only a few other foods. It's a myth that fish is expensive or hard to cook, and we plan to prove it to you in chapter 8.

Poultry, eggs, cheese, and yogurt: As we get closer to the tip of the pyramid, you'll find foods that are eaten often but in smaller amounts. Poultry is eaten in smaller portions than seafood but more often than red meat. Eggs are an inexpensive complete protein source and one of the few natural sources of immune-strengthening vitamin D and brain-boosting choline. Other regular protein staples include yogurt and cheese, which contain calcium and potassium—crucial for bone health—along with probiotics, which help strengthen the immune system.

FOODS TO ENJOY IN MODERATION

At the tip of the pyramid, you'll see the words "less often" next to meats and sweets, which means they are eaten only occasionally.

Red meat: Red meat provides important nutrients, including iron, vitamin B12, and protein, but eating other protein sources such as fish, beans, or nuts often or in place of red meat can lower your risk for several diseases and premature death, and based on a 2012 study in the Archives of Internal Medicine. So eat red meat in smaller amounts, rather like a side dish.

Sweets: Cakes, cookies, ice cream, candies, and pastries are reserved for holidays and celebrations in the Mediterranean Diet. We suggest a gradual approach in cutting back on sweets. Start with fruit for dessert twice a week while reducing portion sizes of baked goods. And don't worry; we have an entire chapter of better-for-you desserts in this book.

Wine: Wine is an integral part of the Mediterranean Diet and should be sipped slowly to enhance the taste and enjoyment of food. In accordance with the current edition of Dietary Guidelines for Americans, subtle drinks are known as two 5-ounce glasses of wine a day for men and one glass for women. These amounts appear to have the most health benefits with the least risks.

FOODS TO CUT BACK ON

Processed meats: Our big beef with processed meats like deli meats, salami, sausage, and bacon is the amount of salt and fillers in them. Cured meats like prosciutto are preferred but are eaten in small amounts and not every day.

Added sugars: We're not talking about naturally occurring sugars in fruits, vegetables, and dairy foods, but rather sugars added to a product. They are lurking everywhere these days—in condiments, yogurts, bread, and drinks—and you may not realize how much you are consuming. Look for "added sugars" on food labels. And in any recipe (not in this book), you can usually decrease the sugar by a few tablespoons. Honey is a traditional sweetener when eating the Mediterranean way, but remember, it's still considered an added sugar.

Refined grains: Refined grains are stripped of the bran and germ during milling, and as a result, the majority of available dietary fiber, iron, B vitamins, and phytonutrients are also removed. They're often found in granola bars, bread, desserts, some cereals, and sweet or savory snacks. They're listed on food labels as wheat flour, rice flour, and any flour or grain without the word "whole" in front of it (except oats, which are always a whole grain).

Sodium: The majority of the sodium in our diets doesn't come from the salt shaker, but rather, from processed foods like frozen dinners, frozen pizzas, fast food, processed meats, and condiments. Look for no-salt-added or lower-sodium labels on canned foods when buying things like tomatoes, beans, and broth. As for table salt, we use kosher or sea salt in our recipes because the granules are bigger, so you use less per recipe, but a little salt is important when cooking to make the other flavors in your recipe shine.

Empty-calorie beverages: Sports drinks, energy drinks, sweetened iced teas, and sodas add only calories and sugar to your diet. Bottom line: Drink water. (And the occasional glass of wine—and we'll give you your coffee, too!)

CHAPTER 4

THE MEDITERRANEAN KITCHEN

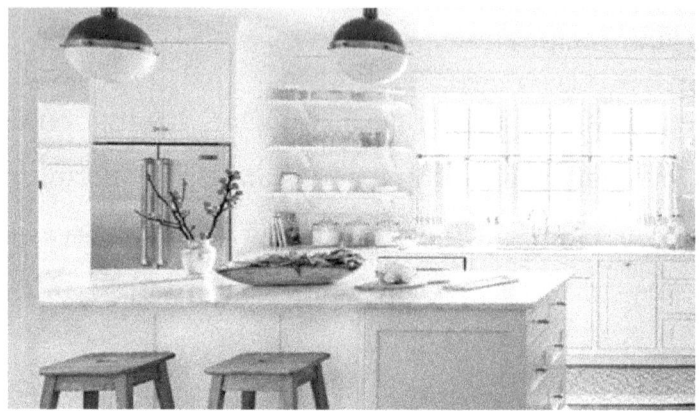

You may already have a Mediterranean kitchen and not even know it. There's no need to buy a lot of expensive ingredients, like many Mediterranean staples, like beans, canned tomatoes, and tuna, are probably in your pantry right now.

Pantry Essentials

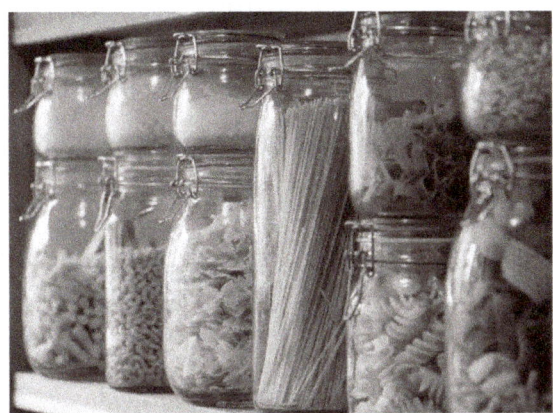

Olives: If your grocery store has an olive bar (often near the deli department), sample different varieties to find your favorites. Then buy that variety in a jar, as they are usually less expensive than at the olive bar. Start tossing olives into soups, salads, sandwiches, pasta, potatoes, or almost any dish in which you'd use salt.

Beans (canned and dried): You can feed a crowd of 10 with one bag of dried beans, which costs about $1.50. Get in the habit of cooking up one batch a week. Dried lentils cook even faster. You also can't go wrong with any can of beans; drain and rinse them to remove about 40 percent of the sodium.

Nuts and seeds: Go nuts over seeds and nuts. Sprinkle a tablespoon or two over any dish to add flavor, crunch, and a dose of good fats. Almonds, pecans, peanuts, pistachios, walnuts, chia seeds, ground flaxseed, pumpkin seeds, and sesame seeds are all nutrition boosters.

Whole grains and brown rice: Whole grains are the foundation of the Mediterranean Diet. Luckily, delicious whole grains like sorghum, quinoa, spelled, and farro are now easier to find. To begin to enjoy whole grains you might be unfamiliar with, combine the new whole grain with rice.

Pasta: Pasta is healthy, low-glycemic-index food. (The glycemic index rates how fast a carbohydrate-rich food is digested and affects your blood sugar levels.) The way dried pasta is made reduces its glycemic index. To get more fiber in your diet, choose whole-grain pasta more often.

Canned fish: We serve budget-friendly canned tuna or salmon a couple of times a week. (Go for the kind packed in olive oil for extra flavor.) Drain sardines or anchovies and mash into tomato sauce for extra nutrients and richness.

Canned and jarred vegetables: Canned, no-salt tomato products are a pantry necessity—especially because the tomato season is short in most parts of the world. Jarred roasted bell peppers, artichoke hearts, and capers are veggie staples you can use daily while eating the Mediterranean way.

Olive oil and vinegar: If you have these two staples on hand, you can flavor any dish (Deanna has 8 to 10 bottles in her pantry!).

We like to use extra-virgin olive oil for cooking and drizzling. It has the most health benefits, and a high enough smoke point to be practical when sautéing. Balsamic vinegar and red wine vinegar are two of our favorites and are typical staples in the Mediterranean Diet.

Kosher or sea salt: You might be surprised to see salt on two dietitians' pantry lists, but remember that the majority of sodium in our diets doesn't come from table salt. That said, the larger grains of these salts means there's less in your measuring spoon, but they still deliver a big flavor punch to dishes.

Grocery Store Guide: How To Shop

Don't follow the old rule that you should only shop the perimeter of the grocery store. Today's supermarkets have Mediterranean Diet staples in every aisle—including the middle ones. While shopping, picture the Mediterranean Diet Pyramid inside your shopping cart: Half your cart should be fruits, vegetables, and plant-based foods, then fill up the rest with seafood, and so on.

Fresh produce section: What's in season? Seasonal fruits and vegetables are usually less expensive. Don't forget fresh herbs: parsley, cilantro, basil, and mint can be budget-friendly ways to eat more always-in-season greens.

Fish counter: Ask questions. The fishmonger behind the counter is happy to steer you to inexpensive choices; he or she can also be a great source for recipes and cooking tips.

Canned fish aisle: There are lots of new additions here, including packets of tuna and salmon that are ready to eat with a fork. Most of the choices are simple and sustainable. Just pick your favorite or try something new, like sardines.

Frozen food aisle: The frozen food aisle is an ideal place to finish filling your cart with fruit and veggies. In general, frozen fruits and vegetables are just as nutritious as fresh, as they are frozen at the peak of freshness. Choose any vegetable without sauce. We buy frozen fruits to go into every breakfast, from cereal to yogurt. Frozen fish fillets are healthy, convenient choices, and because they're often frozen individually, you can cook just what you need.

Rice and grains aisle: In general, you'll find most whole grains here, in the natural foods aisle, or the bulk food section. To make sure the grains are whole, search for these words on the Nutrition Facts label: oats, bulgur, wheat berries, rye berries, or whole [name of grain], such as whole wheat. Look for farro, bulgur, quinoa, sorghum, spelled, barley, brown rice (instant and regular), and wild rice without any added flavors or seasonings.

Bulk food section: This area, with foods in open bins, makes food shopping fun. Here's where you can buy small amounts of things to taste, without spending a lot on full packages of whole grains, beans, and dried fruits.

Dairy case: From low-fat to full-fat, we promote eating the type of milk, cheese, or yogurt that you prefer. Products with more fat will have more calories, but we find that they are more filling and flavorful, and often you can use less in a recipe. When it comes to yogurt, we prefer plain, but if you are buying flavored yogurt, compare the amount of added sugar to other flavored yogurt and go with the lowest number. (The total sugar amount on the label also includes the lactose and fructose—those naturally occurring sugars found in dairy and fruit.) Or better yet, buy the plain and add your fruit.

CHAPTER 5

31 MEAL PLANS (EASY TO PREPARE)

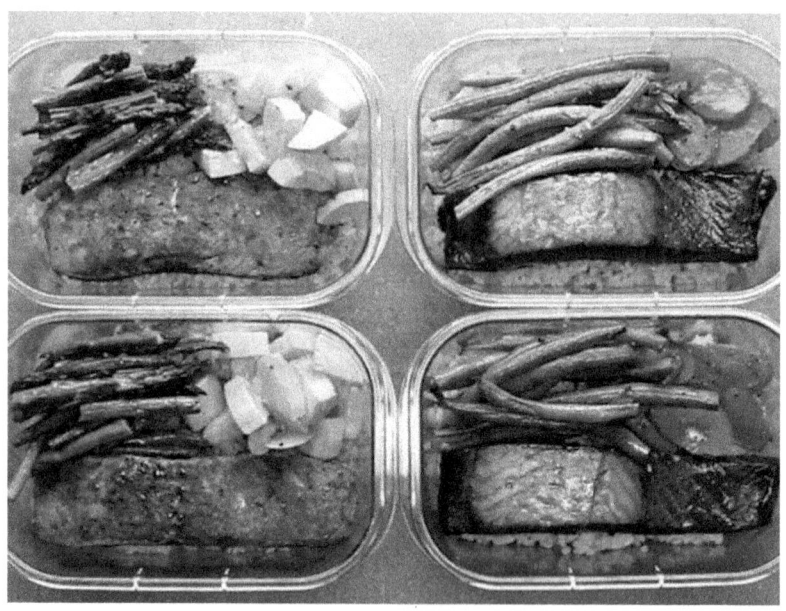

The Mediterranean diet is meant to be followed long term; therefore, the meal plan given in this chapter is designed to help you kickstart your journey. The meal plan was created with the 100 recipes listed in the books. The recipes are flexible and can be rotated among the days as you please.

This is the beginning of your journey, note that you will need a lot of discipline and dedication to continue after the 31 days planned for you. That is when the spirit of diversity and experimentation has to come in. You have to be able to search for dishes online and combine a couple of them to make your very own recipes. Do not isolate yourself to just the 100 recipes listed in this book; there are thousands more on the internet. These are just to get you started.

The recipes listed in this book are all made from fresh, natural, unprocessed foods. Pay attention to the nutritional values given for each dish and use them to plan your meals. Also, don't forget to combine your diet with physical activities and exercise for optimal weight and health.

Bon Appetit!

WEEK 1

Day 1

Breakfast: Oatmeal with Yogurt and Egg

Lunch: Broccolini Almond Pizza

Dinner: Mediterranean Stuffed Chicken Breasts

Day 2

Breakfast: Baked Eggs with Spinach

Lunch: Greek Bruschetta

Dinner: Mediterranean Grilled Chicken Kebabs

Day 3

Breakfast: Quinoa and Dried Fruit

Lunch: Greek Orzo Salad

Dinner: Mediterranean Chicken Couscous

Day 4

Breakfast: Veggie Breakfast Bowl

Lunch: Mediterranean Egg Salad

Dinner: Lemon-Garlic Shrimp

Day 5

Breakfast: Apple Peanut Butter Oatmeal

Lunch: Mediterranean Quinoa Salad

Dinner: Seafood Linguine

Day 6

Breakfast: Edamame and Sweet Pea Hummus

Lunch: Mexican Tuna Salad

Dinner: Seared Salmon and White Beans

Day 7

Breakfast: Eggs and Hash and Cheese

Lunch: Spinach and Tuna Salad

Dinner: Grilled Steak and Sweet Potatoes

Dessert: Chilled Dark Chocolate Fruit Kebabs

WEEK 2

Day 8

Breakfast: Muffin Pan Frittatas

Lunch: Tuscan Style Tuna Salad

Dinner: Baked Lasagna

Day 9

Breakfast: Avacado and Egg Breakfast Sandwich

Lunch: Chicken Souvlaki with Tzatziki

Dinner: Gnocchi, Tomatoes, and Pancetta

Day 10

Breakfast: Mediterranean Frittatas

Lunch: Creamy Paninis

Dinner: Penne and Chicken

Day 11

Breakfast: Mediterranean Breakfast Sandwich

Lunch: Pressed Picnic Sandwich

Dinner: Spinach and Feta Pita Bake

Day 12

Breakfast: Mediterranean Breakfast Wrap

Lunch: Roasted Peppers with Broiled Feta and Olives

Dinner: Mediterranean Flounder

Day 13

Breakfast: Mediterranean Egg Scramble

Lunch: Honey Almond Crusted Chicken Tenders

Dinner: Chicken Costa Brava

Day 14

Breakfast: Breakfast Couscous

Lunch: Spinach with Garbanzo Beans

Dinner: Salmon Panzanella

Dessert: Vanilla Greek Yogurt Affogato

WEEK 3

Day 15

Breakfast: Pomegranate Cherry Smoothie Bowl

Lunch: Grilled Oregano Chicken Kebabs with Zucchini and Olives

Dinner: Stuffed Sardines

Day 16

Breakfast: Greek Yogurt Breakfast Parfaits with Roasted Grapes

Lunch: One-Pan Parsley Chicken and Potatoes

Dinner: Mini Greek Meatloaves

Day 17

Breakfast: Mashed Chickpea, Feta, and Avocado Toast

Lunch: Romesco Poached Chicken

Dinner: Yogurt-and-Herb Marinated Pork Tenderloin

Day 18

Breakfast: Quickie Honey Nut Granola

Lunch: Roasted Red Pepper Chicken with Lemony Garlic Hummus

Dinner: Turkish Lamb Stew

Day 19

Breakfast: Breakfast Polenta

Lunch: Moroccan Meatballs

Dinner: Speedy Tilapia with Red Onion and Avocado

Day 20

Breakfast: Baked Ricotta with Pears

Lunch: Beef Spanakopita Pita Pockets

Dinner: Grilled Fish on Lemons

Day 21

Breakfast: Mediterranean Fruit Bulgur Breakfast Bowl

Lunch: Grilled Steak, Mushroom, and Onion Kebabs

Dinner: Weeknight Sheet Pan Fish Dinner

Dessert: Grilled Stone Fruit with Whipped Ricotta

WEEK 4

Day 22

Breakfast: Scrambled Eggs with Goat Cheese and Roasted Peppers

Lunch: Beef Gyros with Tahini Sauce

Dinner: Crispy Polenta Fish Sticks

Day 23

Breakfast: Marinara Eggs with Parsley

Lunch: Beef Sliders with Pepper Slaw

Dinner: Greek Stuffed Collard Greens

Day 24

Breakfast: Italian Breakfast Bruschetta

Lunch: Shrimp Scampi

Dinner: Walnut Pesto Zoodles

Day 25

Breakfast: Julene's Green Juice

Lunch: Shrimp Mojo de Ajo

Dinner: Cauliflower Steaks with Eggplant Relish

Day 26

Breakfast: Chocolate Banana Smoothie

Lunch: Pan-Seared Scallops with Sautéed Spinach

Dinner: East Brussel Sprouts Hash

Day 27

Breakfast: Fruit Smoothie

Lunch: Pasta Puttanesca

Dinner: Roasted Asparagus with Lemon and Pine Nuts

Day 28

Breakfast: Berry and Yogurt Parfait

Lunch: Pasta with Pesto

Dinner: Citrus Sautéed Spinach

Dessert: Pomegranate-Quinoa Dark Chocolate Bark

WEEK 5

Day 29

Breakfast: Yogurt with Blueberries, Honey, and Mint

Lunch: Greek Meatballs (Keftedes)

Dinner: Mashed Cauliflower

Day 30

Breakfast: Almond and Maple Quick Grits

Lunch: Lamb with String Beans (Arni Me Fasolakia)

Dinner: Broccoli with Ginger and Garlic

Day 31

Breakfast: Oatmeal with Berries and Sunflower Seeds

Lunch: Shrimp Scampi

Dinner: Balsamic Roasted Carrots

Dessert: Lemon Fool

CHAPTER 6

BREAKFAST RECIPES

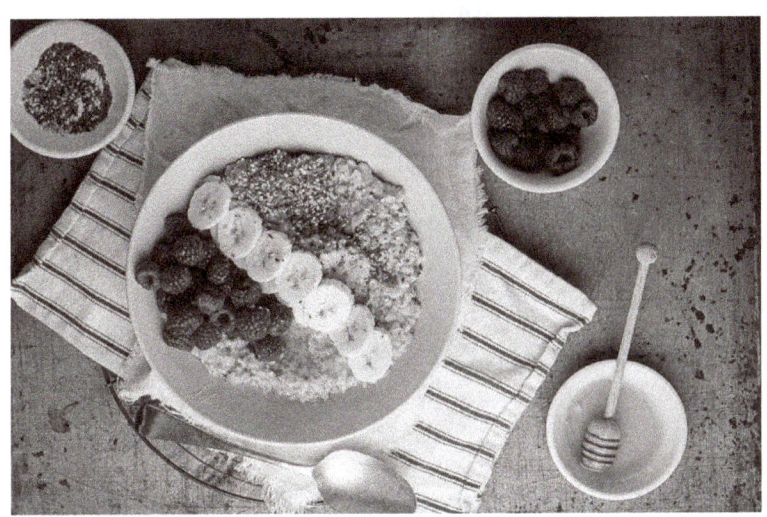

01. Oatmeal With Yogurt & Egg

Preparation Time: 5 minutes
Cooking Time: 2 minutes
Servings: 1

Ingredients:

- ⅓ c. oats
- ⅓ c. low-fat milk
- 1 egg
- ¼ tsp. cinnamon
- ¼ c. yogurt
- ¼ c. slashed apple
- Salt
- Sugar

Directions:

1. Blend the milk and egg. Mix in all ingredients except yogurt and apple.

2. Microwave until the liquid is evaporated, (for about 2 minutes).

3. Spread yogurt and apples on top of oatmeal.

Nutrition:

320 calories

46g Carbs

9g fat

17g protein

02. Baked Eggs With Spinach

Preparation Time: 5 minutes

Cooking Time: 20 minutes

Servings: 4

Ingredients:

- 4 eggs

- 1 package frozen spinach

- ¼ c. shredded Cheddar cheese

- ¼ c. chunky salsa

Directions:

1. Preheat oven to 325°F.

2. Put an equal amount of spinach into 4 custard cups. Make a well in the middle by pressing down with your fingers.

3. Add an egg into each indentation. Spoon salsa and shredded

cheese on the top.

4. Cook for 20 min.

Nutrition:

120 calories

4g carbs

7g fat

10g protein

03. Quinoa & Dried Fruit

Preparation Time: 10 minutes
Cooking Time: 15 minutes
Servings: 4

Ingredients:

- 3 c. water

- 1 c. quinoa

- ¼ c. walnuts

- 8 dried apricots

- 4 dried figs

- 1 tsp. cinnamon

Directions:

1. In a pot, mix water and quinoa and let simmer for 15 minutes, until the water evaporates.

2. Chop dried fruit.

3. When quinoa is cooked, stir in all other ingredients.

4. Serve cold. Add milk, if desired.

Nutrition:

44g carbs
7g fat
13g protein
285 calories

04. Eggs & Hash & Cheese

Preparation Time: 5 minutes
Cooking Time: 2 minutes
Servings: 1

Ingredients:

- 1 egg

- ½ c. shredded hash browns

- 2 tbsps. cheddar cheese

- Salt

- Pepper

Directions:

1. Grease a microwaveable bowl with olive oil spray and fill with hashbrowns. Microwave for 1 minute, and add salt and pepper to taste.

2. Stir in an egg and beat well. Microwave for 45 seconds.

3. Sprinkle cheese over the top.

Nutrition:

7g carbs

14g fat

15g protein

210 calories

05. Veggie Breakfast Bowl

Preparation Time: 5 minutes

Cooking Time: 2 minutes

Servings: 1

Ingredients:

- 1 egg
- 1 tbsp. water
- 2 tbsps. shredded mozzarella cheese
- 2 tbsps. diced mushrooms
- ¼ c. baby spinach
- 2 tbsps. cherry tomatoes

Directions:

1. Mix all ingredients excluding the cheese

in a greased microwaveable bowl.

2. Microwave for 1 minute or until the egg is cooked.

3. Sprinkle shredded cheese over the top.

Nutrition:

2g carbs

6g fat

10g protein

100 calories

06. Apple Peanut Butter Oatmeal

Preparation Time: 15 minutes

Cooking Time: 8 hours

Servings: 4

Ingredients:

- 1 c. steel-cut oats
- ¼ c. brown sugar
- ½ tsp. cinnamon
- ¼ c. peanut butter
- 1 tsp. vanilla extract
- 2 diced apples
- Salt

Directions:

1. Grease a slow cooker with cooking spray.

2. Add all ingredients to the crockpot except apples, mix well.

3. Add apples to the top of the mixture and cook on low for 8 hours.

Nutrition:

50g carbs

11g fat

10g protein

320 calories

07. Edamame & Sweet Pea Hummus

Preparation Time: 5 minutes

Cooking Time: 2 minutes

Servings: 2

Ingredients:

- ½ c. edamame

- ½ c. peas

- 2 tbsps. Tahini

- 1 minced garlic clove

- 2 tbsps. chopped mint

- 3 tbsps. olive oil

- 2 wheat tortillas

- 2 eggs

Directions:

1. Blend the first 5 ingredients and 1 Tbsp. of olive oil in a food processor. Spread evenly over the wheat tortillas.

2. Coat pan with remaining olive oil and cook the eggs. When ready, put one egg on each tortilla.

Nutrition:

35g carbs

30g fat

20g protein

460 calories

08. Muffin Pan Frittatas

Preparation Time: 10 minutes

Cooking Time: 15 minutes

Servings: 6

Ingredients:

- 6 eggs

- ½ c. milk

- 1 c. cheddar cheese

- ¾ c. chopped zucchini

- ¼ c. chopped red bell pepper

- 2 tbsps. sliced red onion

- Pepper

Directions:

1. Preheat oven to 350°F.

2. Mix the milk, eggs, and pepper. Then mix in other ingredients.

3. Spray cooking spray on a muffin tin and distribute the prepared mixture evenly between the cups. Bake for 15 min.

Nutrition:

3g carbs

10g fat

12g protein

165 calories

09. Avocado & Egg Breakfast Sandwich

Preparation Time: 5 minutes

Cooking Time: 5 minutes

Servings: 2

Ingredients:

- 4 toasted bread slices

- 1 avocado

- 12 steamed asparagus spears

- 1 sliced hard-boiled egg

- Olive oil

- Pepper

- Sea salt

- Dijon mustard

Directions:

1. Peel and mash the avocado and toast the bread.

2. Prepare the sandwich by using the mustard with a layer of the avocado.

3. Add the asparagus spears and eggs. Give it a drizzle of oil along with some salt and pepper. Close and enjoy.

Nutrition:

283.6 calories
11.5g fat
31g carbs
10.9g protein

10.   Mediterranean Frittata

Preparation Time: 10 minutes
Cooking Time: 15-20 minutes
Servings: 6

Ingredients:

- ½ c. diced tomatoes

- ½ c. milk

- 6 eggs

- ¼ c. of each

- ¼ c. Kalamata

- 1 c. chopped spinach

- ½ tsp. pepper

- 1 tsp. oregano

- 1 tsp. salt

- ¼ c. crumbled feta

Directions:

1. Program the oven temperature to 400ºF.

2. Grease the chosen dish, and whisk the milk and eggs.

3. Combine all of the fixings, mixing well.

4. Bake for 15-20 minutes. The eggs will be set and ready to serve.

Nutrition:

242 Calories

7g Carbs

19g Fat

12g Protein

11.   Mediterranean Breakfast Sandwich

Preparation Time: 5 minutes

Cooking Time: 5 minutes

Servings: 1

Ingredients:

- 1 Heirloom Tomato

- 1 Onion

- 2 slices of Bread

- ¼ Zucchini

- 1 Egg

- 1 tbsp. Basil

- Salt

Directions:

1. Begin by thinly slicing the onion, zucchini, tomato, and basil leaves.

2. Place the olive oil into the pan on medium heat and add an egg. The style of the egg is up to you.

3. Meanwhile, toast your bread slices in a toaster.

4. Place one slice of bread onto a plate and lay the egg on top.

5. In the pan, set the zucchini and onion and allow them to brown. This should take only a few minutes.

6. On the other slice of bread, layer your tomato and basil.

7. Once your onion and zucchini are soft, layer them on top of the tomato and basil.

8. Finally, layer the bread pieces on top of one another and your sandwich is complete!

Nutrition:

242 calories

25g carbs

12g fat

13g protein

12.   Mediterranean Breakfast Wrap

Preparation Time: 10

minutes

Cooking Time: 10 minutes

Servings: 2

Ingredients:

- ¼ c. red pepper

- ¼ c. onion

- 1 tomato

- ½ c. baby spinach

- 1 c. egg substitute

- 1½ tsps. fresh basil

- 2 wheat tortillas

- 2 tbsps. feta cheese

- 1 tbsp. olive oil

Directions:

1. Begin by heating the olive oil into your pan and then add your pepper and onion.

2. Continue cooking the onion and pepper over medium heat until soft.

3. Next, add the egg substitute with the spices and cook until eggs are as desired.

4. Once the egg is cooked, you will want to place the spinach, tomato, and egg into the wrap.

5. Add the crumbled feta cheese onto the wrap, and your meal is complete!

Nutrition:

448 calories

27g fat

41g carbs

15g protein

13. Mediterranean Egg Scramble

Preparation Time: 10 minutes
Cooking Time: 15 minutes
Servings: 4

Ingredients:

- 4 Slices bread

- 6 Eggs

- ¼ diced red bell pepper

- 3 sliced potatoes

- 8 chopped black olives

- ¼ c. fresh ricotta cheese

- ¼ c. parsley

- 5 tsp. butter

- 1 tsp. olive oil

Directions:

1. Begin by heating the olive oil and butter in a pan over medium-high heat.

2. Once the olive oil and butter are simmering, add the sliced potatoes into the pan and sauté for 15 minutes.

3. Once potatoes are golden, add the bell pepper and olives. Allow these to cook for about 4 minutes.

4. When this mixture is complete, take a medium bowl and whisk your eggs, ricotta, and parsley together.

5. In your pan, you will

want to pour the egg mixture over the potato mixture.

6. Stir the mixture every 30 seconds so that the mixture is firm but not dry. Do this for about 3 minutes.

7. Once the mixture is complete, place it over your toasted bread, and your meal is complete!

Nutrition:

324 Calories

24g fat

20g protein

7g carbs

14. Breakfast Couscous

Preparation Time: 10 minutes
Cooking Time: 15 minutes
Servings: 4

Ingredients:

- 1 c. uncooked whole-wheat couscous

- 3 c. low-fat milk

- ½ c. currants, dried

- 1 (2 in.) cinnamon stick

- ½ c. apricots, dried

- ¼ tsp. salt

- 6 tsp. dark brown sugar, divided

- 4 tsp. melted butter divided

Directions:

1. Using a medium-high burner on the stovetop, place a large saucepan and add the cinnamon stick and milk. Heat it until you see bubble formations along the edges. (Do not bring to a boil.)

2. Remove the pan from the burner and blend in the apricots, couscous, salt, currants, and four teaspoons of the brown sugar.

3. Close the lid and let it rest for 15 minutes. Take the top off and throw away the cinnamon stick.

4. Serve evenly in four bowls and garnish with the rest of the brown sugar and a teaspoon of melted butter.

Nutrition:

306 calories

6g fat

55g carbs

11g protein

15. Pomegranate Cherry Smoothie Bowl

Preparation Time: 5 minutes

Cooking Time: 0 minutes

Servings: 4

Ingredients:

- 1 (16-ounce) bag frozen dark sweet cherries

- 1½ cups 2% plain Greek yogurt, plus more if needed

- ¾ cup pomegranate juice

- ⅓ cup 2% milk, plus more if needed

- 1 teaspoon vanilla extract

- ¾ teaspoon ground cinnamon

- 6 ice cubes

- ½ cup chopped pistachios

- ½ cup fresh pomegranate seeds

Directions:

1. Put the cherries, yogurt, pomegranate juice, milk, vanilla, cinnamon, and ice cubes in a blender. Purée until thoroughly mixed and smooth. You'll want the mixture a little thicker than your average smoothie, but not so thick you can't pour it. If the smoothie is too thick, add another few tablespoons of milk; if it's too thin, add another few tablespoons of yogurt.

2. Pour the smoothie into four bowls. Top each with 2 tablespoons of pistachios and 2 tablespoons of pomegranate seeds, and serve

immediately.

Nutrition:

Calories: 212

Total Fat: 7g

Saturated Fat: 3g

Cholesterol: 18mg

Sodium: 53mg

Total Carbohydrates: 35g

Fiber: 3g

Protein: 4g

16. Greek Yogurt Breakfast Parfaits With Roasted Grapes

Preparation Time: 5 minutes

Cooking Time: 25 minutes

Servings: 4

Ingredients:

- 1½ pounds seedless grapes (about 4 cups)

- 1 tablespoon extra-virgin olive oil

- 2 cups 2% plain Greek yogurt

- ½ cup chopped walnuts

- 4 teaspoons honey

Directions:

1. Place a large, rimmed baking sheet in the oven. Preheat the oven to 450°F with the pan inside.

2. Wash the grapes and remove them from the stems. Dry on a clean kitchen towel, and put in a bowl. Drizzle with the oil, and toss to coat.

3. Carefully remove the hot pan from the

oven, and pour the grapes onto the pan. Bake for 20 to 23 minutes, until slightly shriveled, stirring once halfway through. Remove the baking sheet from the oven and cool on a wire rack for 5 minutes.

4. While the grapes are cooling, assemble the parfaits by spooning the yogurt into four bowls or tall glasses. Top each bowl or glass with 2 tablespoons of walnuts and 1 teaspoon of honey.

5. When the grapes are slightly cooled, top each parfait with a quarter of the grapes. Scrape any accumulated sweet grape juice onto the parfaits and serve.

Nutrition:

Calories: 300

Total Fat: 17g

Saturated Fat: 4g

Cholesterol: 16mg

Sodium: 59mg

Total Carbohydrates: 34g

Fiber: 2g

Protein: 7g

17. Mashed Chickpea, Feta, And Avocado Toast

Preparation Time: 10 minutes

Cooking Time: 0 minutes

Servings: 4

Ingredients:

- 1 (15-ounce) can chickpeas, drained and rinsed

- 1 avocado, pitted

- ½ cup diced feta cheese (about 2 ounces)

- 2 teaspoons freshly squeezed lemon juice or 1 tablespoon orange juice

- ½ teaspoon freshly ground black pepper

- 4 pieces multigrain toast

- 2 teaspoons honey

Directions:

1. Put the chickpeas in a large bowl. Scoop the avocado flesh into the bowl.

2. With a potato masher or large fork, mash the ingredients together until the mix has a spreadable consistency. It doesn't need to be totally smooth.

3. Add the feta, lemon juice, and pepper, and mix well.

4. Evenly divide the mash onto the four pieces of toast and spread with a knife. Drizzle with honey and serve.

Nutrition:

Calories: 337

Total Fat: 13g

Saturated Fat: 4g

Cholesterol: 16mg

Sodium: 564mg

Total Carbohydrates: 43g

Fiber: 12g

Protein: 13g

18. Quickie Honey Nut Granola

Preparation Time: 10 minutes

Cooking Time: 20 minutes

Servings: 6

Ingredients:

- 2½ cups regular rolled oats

- ⅓ cup coarsely chopped almonds

- ⅛ teaspoon kosher or sea salt

- ½ teaspoon ground cinnamon

- ½ cup chopped dried apricots

- 2 tablespoons ground flaxseed

- ¼ cup honey

- ¼ cup extra-virgin olive oil

- 2 teaspoons vanilla extract

Directions:

1. Preheat the oven to 325°F. Line a large, rimmed baking sheet with parchment paper.

2. In a large skillet, combine the oats, almonds, salt, and cinnamon. Turn the heat to medium-high and cook, stirring often, to toast, about 6 minutes.

3. While the oat

mixture is toasting, in a microwave-safe bowl, combine the apricots, flaxseed, honey, and oil. Microwave on high for about 1 minute, or until very hot and just beginning to bubble. (Or heat these ingredients in a small saucepan over medium heat for about 3 minutes.)

4. Stir the vanilla into the honey mixture, then pour it over the oat mixture in the skillet. Stir well.

5. Spread out the granola on the prepared baking sheet. Bake for 15 minutes, until lightly browned. Remove from the oven and cool completely.

6. Break the granola into small pieces, and store in an airtight container in the refrigerator for up to 2 weeks (if it lasts that long!).

Nutrition:

Calories: 337

Total Fat: 17g

Saturated Fat: 2g

Cholesterol: 0mg

Sodium: 23mg

Total Carbohydrates: 42g

Fiber: 6g

Protein: 7g

19. Breakfast Polenta

Preparation Time: 5 minutes

Cooking Time: 10 minutes

Servings: 6

Ingredients:

- 2 (18-ounce) tubes plain polenta

- 2¼ to 2½ cups 2% milk, divided

- 2 oranges, peeled and chopped

- ½ cup chopped pecans

- ¼ cup 2% plain Greek yogurt

- 8 teaspoons honey

Directions:

- Slice the polenta into rounds and place in a microwave-safe bowl. Heat in the microwave on high for 45 seconds.

- Transfer the polenta to a large pot, and mash it with a potato masher or fork until coarsely mashed. Place the pot on the stove over medium heat.

- In a medium, microwave-safe bowl, heat the milk in the microwave on high for 1 minute. Pour 2 cups of the warmed milk into the pot with the polenta, and stir with a whisk. Continue to stir and mash with the whisk, adding the remaining milk a few tablespoons at a time, until the polenta is fairly smooth and heated through about 5 minutes. Remove from the stove.

- Divide the polenta among four serving bowls. Top each bowl with one-quarter of the oranges, 2 tablespoons of pecans, 1 tablespoon of yogurt, and 2 teaspoons of honey before serving.

Nutrition:

Calories: 234

Total Fat: 7g

Saturated Fat: 2g

Cholesterol: 5mg

Sodium: 438mg

Total Carbohydrates: 38mg

Fiber: 4g

Protein: 3g

20. Baked Ricotta With Pears

Preparation Time: 5 minutes

Cooking Time: 25 minutes

Servings: 4

Ingredients:

- Nonstick cooking spray

- 1 (16-ounce) container whole-milk ricotta cheese

- 2 large eggs

- ¼ cup white whole-wheat flour or whole-wheat pastry flour

- 1 tablespoon sugar

- 1 teaspoon vanilla extract

- ¼ teaspoon ground nutmeg

- 1 pear, cored and diced

- 2 tablespoons water

- 1 tablespoon honey

Directions:

1. Preheat the oven to 400°F. Spray four 6-ounce ramekins with nonstick cooking spray.

2. In a large bowl, beat together the ricotta, eggs, flour, sugar, vanilla, and nutmeg. Spoon into the ramekins. Bake for 22 to 25 minutes, or until the ricotta is just about set. Remove from the oven and cool slightly on racks.

3. While the ricotta is baking, in a small saucepan over medium heat, simmer the pear in the water for 10 minutes, until slightly softened. Remove from the heat, and stir in the honey.

4. Serve the ricotta ramekins topped with the warmed pear.

Nutrition:

Calories: 312

Total Fat: 17g

Saturated Fat: 10g

Cholesterol: 163mg

Sodium: 130mg

Total Carbohydrates: 23g

Fiber: 2g

Protein: 17g

21. Mediterranean Fruit Bulgur Breakfast Bowl

Preparation Time: 5 minutes

Cooking Time: 15 minutes

Servings: 6

Ingredients:

- 1½ cups uncooked bulgur

- 2 cups 2% milk

- 1 cup of water

- ½ teaspoon ground cinnamon

- 2 cups frozen (or fresh, pitted) dark sweet cherries

- 8 dried (or fresh) figs, chopped

- ½ cup chopped almonds

- ¼ cup loosely packed fresh mint, chopped

- Warm 2% milk, for serving (optional)

Directions:

1. In a medium saucepan, combine the bulgur, milk, water, and cinnamon. Stir once, then bring just to a boil. Cover, reduce the heat to medium-low, and simmer for 10 minutes or until the liquid is absorbed.

2. Turn off the heat, but keep the pan on the stove, and stir in the frozen cherries (no need to thaw), figs, and almonds. Stir well, cover for 1 minute, and let the hot bulgur thaw the cherries and partially hydrate the figs. Stir in the mint.

3. Scoop into serving bowls. Serve with warm milk, if desired. You can also serve it chilled.

Nutrition:

Calories: 301
Total Fat: 6g
Saturated Fat: 1g
Cholesterol: 7mg
Sodium: 40mg
Total Carbohydrates: 57g

Fiber: 9g
Protein: 9g

22. Scrambled Eggs With Goat Cheese And Roasted Peppers

Preparation Time: 5 minutes
Cooking Time: 10 minutes
Servings: 4

Ingredients:

- 1½ teaspoons extra-virgin olive oil

- 1 cup chopped bell peppers, any color (about 1 medium pepper)

- 2 garlic cloves, minced (about 1 teaspoon)

- 6 large eggs

- ¼ teaspoon kosher or sea salt

- 2 tablespoons water

- ½ cup crumbled goat cheese (about 2 ounces)

- 2 tablespoons loosely packed chopped fresh mint

Directions:

1. In a large skillet over medium-high heat, heat the oil. Add the peppers and cook for 5 minutes, stirring occasionally. Add the garlic and cook for 1 minute.

2. While the peppers are cooking, in a medium bowl, whisk together the eggs, salt, and water.

3. Turn the heat down to medium-low. Pour the egg mixture over the peppers. Let the eggs cook undisturbed for 1 to 2 minutes until they begin to set on the bottom. Sprinkle with the goat cheese.

4. Cook the eggs for about 1 to 2 more minutes, stirring slowly, until the eggs are soft-set and custardy. (They will continue to cook off the stove from the residual heat in the pan.)

5. Top with the fresh mint and serve.

Nutrition:

Calories: 201
Total Fat: 15g
Saturated Fat: 6g
Cholesterol: 294mg
Sodium: 176mg
Total Carbohydrates: 5g
Fiber: 2g
Protein: 15g

23. Marinara Eggs With Parsley

Preparation Time: 5 minutes
Cooking Time: 15 minutes
Servings: 6

Ingredients:

- 1 tablespoon extra-virgin olive oil

- 1 cup chopped onion (about ½ medium onion)

- 2 garlic cloves, minced (about 1 teaspoon)

- 2 (14.5-ounce) cans Italian diced tomatoes, undrained, no salt added

- 6 large eggs

- ½ cup chopped fresh flat-leaf (Italian) parsley

- Crusty Italian bread and grated Parmesan or Romano cheese, for serving (optional)

Directions:

1. In a large skillet over medium-high heat, heat the oil. Add the

onion and cook for 5 minutes, stirring occasionally. Add the garlic and cook for 1 minute.

2. Pour the tomatoes with their juices over the onion mixture and cook until bubbling, 2 to 3 minutes. While waiting for the tomato mixture to bubble, crack one egg into a small custard cup or coffee mug.

3. When the tomato mixture bubbles, lower the heat to medium. Then use a large spoon to make six indentations in the tomato mixture.

Gently pour the first cracked egg into one indentation and repeat, cracking the remaining eggs, one at a time, into the custard cup and pouring one into each indentation. Cover the skillet and cook for 6 to 7 minutes, or until the eggs are done to your liking (about 6 minutes for soft-cooked, 7 minutes for harder cooked).

4. Top with the parsley, and serve with the bread and grated cheese, if desired.

Nutrition:

Calories: 122

Total Fat: 7g

Saturated Fat: 2g

Cholesterol: 186mg

Sodium: 207mg

Total Carbohydrates: 7g

Fiber: 1g

Protein: 7g

24. Italian Breakfast Bruschetta

Preparation Time: 10 minutes

Cooking Time: 20 minutes

Servings: 4

Ingredients:

- ¼ teaspoon kosher or sea salt

- 6 cups broccoli rabe, stemmed and chopped (about 1 bunch)

- 1 tablespoon extra-virgin olive oil

- 2 garlic cloves, minced (about 1 teaspoon)

- 1-ounce prosciutto, cut or torn into ½-inch pieces

- ¼ teaspoon crushed red pepper

- Nonstick cooking spray

- 3 large eggs

- 1 tablespoon 2% milk

- ¼ teaspoon freshly ground black pepper

- 4 teaspoons grated Parmesan or Pecorino Romano cheese

- 1 garlic clove, halved

- 8 (¾-inch-thick)

slices baguette-style whole-grain bread or 4 slices larger Italian-style whole-grain bread

Directions:

1. Bring a large stockpot of water to a boil. Add the salt and broccoli rabe, and boil for 2 minutes. Drain in a colander.

2. In a large skillet over medium heat, heat the oil. Add the garlic, prosciutto, and crushed red pepper, and cook for 2 minutes, stirring often. Add the broccoli rabe and cook for an additional 3 minutes, stirring a few times. Transfer to a bowl and set aside.

3. Place the skillet back on the stove over low heat and coat with nonstick cooking spray.

4. In a small bowl, whisk together the eggs, milk, and pepper. Pour into the skillet. Stir and cook until the eggs are soft-scrambled, 3 to 5 minutes. Add the broccoli rabe mixture back to the skillet along with the cheese. Stir and cook for about 1 minute, until heated through. Remove from the heat.

5. Toast the bread, then rub the cut sides of the garlic clove halves onto one side of each slice of the toast. (Save the garlic for another recipe.) Spoon the egg mixture onto each piece of toast and serve.

Nutrition:

Calories: 216

Total Fat: 9g

Saturated Fat: 2g

Cholesterol: 145mg

Sodium: 522mg

Total Carbohydrates: 20g

Fiber: 5g

Protein: 13g

25. Julene's Green Juice

Preparation Time: 5 minutes

Cooking Time: 0 minutes

Servings: 1

Ingredients:

- 3 cups dark leafy greens

- 1 cucumber

- ¼ cup fresh Italian parsley leaves

- ¼ pineapple, cut into wedges

- ½ green apple

- ½ orange

- ½ lemon

- Pinch grated fresh ginger

Directions:

Using a juicer, run the greens, cucumber, parsley, pineapple, apple, orange,

lemon, and ginger through it, pour into a large cup, and serve.

Nutrition:

Calories: 108
Protein: 11g
Total Carbohydrates: 29g
Sugars: 10g
Fiber: 9g
Total Fat: 2g
Saturated Fat: 0g
Cholesterol: 0mg
Sodium: 119mg

26. Chocolate Banana Smoothie

Preparation Time: 5 minutes
Cooking Time: 0 minutes
Servings: 2

Ingredients:

- 2 bananas, peeled
- 1 cup unsweetened almond milk, or skim milk
- 1 cup crushed ice
- 3 tablespoons unsweetened cocoa powder
- 3 tablespoons honey

Directions:

In a blender, combine the bananas, almond milk, ice, cocoa powder, and honey. Blend until smooth.

Nutrition:

Calories: 219
Protein: 2g
Total Carbohydrates: 57g
Sugars: 40g
Fiber: 6g
Total Fat: 2g
Saturated Fat: <1g
Cholesterol: 0mg

27. Fruit Smoothie

Preparation Time: 5 minutes
Cooking Time: 0 minutes
Servings: 2

Ingredients:

- 2 cups blueberries (or any fresh or frozen fruit, cut into pieces if the fruit is large)

- 2 cups unsweetened almond milk

- 1 cup crushed ice

- ½ teaspoon ground ginger (or other dried ground spice such as turmeric, cinnamon, or nutmeg)

Directions:

1. In a blender, combine the blueberries, almond milk, ice, and ginger. Blend until smooth.

Nutrition:

Calories: 125
Protein: 2g
Total Carbohydrates: 23g
Sugars: 14g
Fiber: 5g
Total Fat: 4g
Saturated Fat: <1g
Cholesterol: 0mg
Sodium: 181mg

28. Berry And Yogurt Parfait

Preparation Time: 5 minutes
Cooking Time: 0 minutes
Servings: 2

Ingredients:

- 1 cup raspberries

- 1½ cups unsweetened nonfat plain Greek yogurt

- 1 cup blackberries

- ¼ cup chopped walnuts

Directions:

In 2 bowls, layer the raspberries, yogurt, and blackberries. Sprinkle with the walnuts.

Nutrition:

Calories: 290
Protein: 29g
Total Carbohydrates: 27g
Sugars: 12g
Fiber: 10g
Total Fat: 10g
Saturated Fat: <1g
Cholesterol: 15mg
Sodium: 92mg

29. Yogurt With Blueberries, Honey, And Mint

Preparation Time: 5 minutes
Cooking Time: 0 minutes
Servings: 2

Ingredients:

- 2 cups unsweetened nonfat plain Greek yogurt

- 1 cup blueberries

- 3 tablespoons honey

- 2 tablespoons fresh mint leaves, chopped

Directions:

Apportion the yogurt between 2 small bowls. Top with the blueberries, honey, and mint.

Nutrition:

Calories: 314

Protein: 15g

Total Carbohydrates: 54g

Sugars: 50g

Fiber: 2g

Total Fat: 3g

Saturated Fat: 3g

Cholesterol: 15mg

Sodium: 175mg

30. Almond And Maple Quick Grits

Preparation Time: 5 minutes

Cooking Time: 6 minutes

Servings: 4

Ingredients:

- 1½ cups water

- ½ cup unsweetened almond milk

- Pinch sea salt

- ½ cup quick-cooking grits

- ½ teaspoon ground cinnamon

- ¼ cup pure maple syrup

- ¼ cup slivered almonds

Directions:

1. In a medium saucepan over medium-high heat, heat the water, almond milk, and sea salt until it boils.

2. Stirring constantly with a wooden spoon, slowly add the grits. Continue stirring to prevent lumps and bring the mixture to a slow boil. Reduce the heat

to medium-low. Simmer for 5 to 6 minutes, stirring frequently, until the water is completely absorbed.

3. Stir in the cinnamon, syrup, and almonds. Cook for 1 minute more, stirring.

Nutrition:

Calories: 151
Protein: 3g
Total Carbohydrates: 28g
Sugars: 12g
Fiber: 3g
Total Fat: 4g
Saturated Fat: <1g
Cholesterol: 0mg
Sodium: 83mg

31. Oatmeal With Berries And Sunflower Seeds

Preparation Time: 5 minutes
Cooking Time: 10 minutes
Servings: 4

Ingredients:

- 1¾ cups water

- ½ cup unsweetened almond milk

- Pinch sea salt

- 1 cup old-fashioned oats

- ½ cup blueberries

- ½ cup raspberries

- ¼ cup sunflower seeds

Directions:

1. In a medium saucepan over medium-high heat, heat the water, almond milk, and sea salt to a boil.

2. Stir in the oats. Reduce the heat to medium-low and cook, stirring occasionally, for 5 minutes. Cover, and let the oatmeal stand for 2 minutes more. Stir and serve topped with the blueberries, raspberries, and sunflower seeds.

Nutrition:

Calories: 186
Protein: 6g
Total Carbohydrates: 32g
Sugars: 4g

Fiber: 5g
Total Fat: 4g
Saturated Fat: <1g
Cholesterol: 0mg
Sodium: 96mg

CHAPTER 7

LUNCH RECIPES

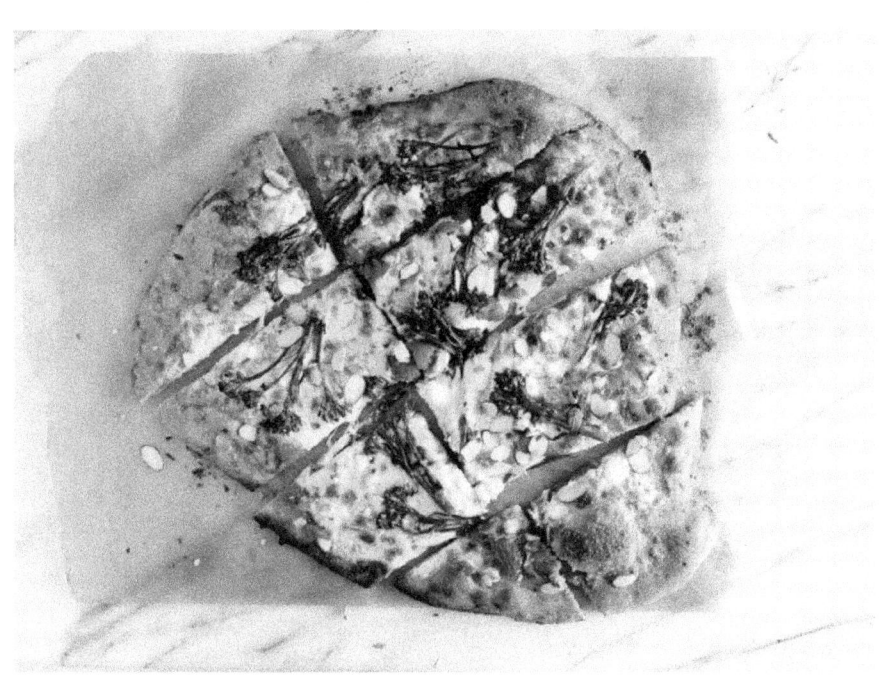

32. Broccolini Almond Pizza

Preparation Time: 10 minutes

Cooking Time: 15 minutes

Servings: 6

Ingredients:

- 1 lb. homemade pizza dough

- 2/3 c. marinara sauce/32 oz. drained & crushed whole tomatoes

- ½ c. crumbled feta

- 8 oz. broccolini

- 2 c. shredded mozzarella cheese

- 1 tsp. EVOO

- ¼ c. sliced almonds

- Basil leaves

- Red pepper flakes

Directions:

1. Set the oven temperature to 500ºF. using the upper third of the oven.

2. Prepare the dough by spreading the sauce over the two pizzas. Add the feta and mozzarella.

3. Prepare the broccolini in a large pot with a few inches of hot water. Trim the ends and add them to the boiling water. Allow to boil and let it steam one minute. Drain and pay them dry.

4. Toss the broccolini into the oil until coated evenly. Add over the pizzas and sprinkle with the almonds. Bake 12 minutes or until done.

5. Slice, garnish as you like, and serve.

Nutrition:

297 calories

12.2g fat

36g carbs

14.3g protein

33. Greek Bruschetta

Preparation Time: 10 minutes

Cooking Time: 15 minutes

Servings: 6

Ingredients:

- 1 tbsp. olive oil

- 1 large garlic clove

- 1 whole-grain baguette

- ¼ c. Chopped fresh basil

- ¼ c. chopped Kalamata olives pitted

- 2 c. cherry tomatoes, quartered

- 1 tbsp. Balsamic vinegar

- 1 tsp. Olive oil

- 1 tsp. dried oregano

- Pinch of pepper

- Pinch of Salt

Directions:

1. Set the oven in advance to 425ºF.

2. Slice the baguette into ½-inch slices. Rub with garlic. Brush with the oil and add in a single layer in a large (with rim) baking tin.

3. Bake five to eight minutes on each side.

4. Meanwhile, mix the ingredients for the bruschetta. Toss to evenly coat and adjust seasonings to your taste.

5. Serve with the tomatoes to the side in a dish. It will keep in the fridge for two days.

6. Enjoy a quick lunch or snack!

Nutrition:

127 calories

7g fat

13g carbs

3g protein

34. Greek Orzo Salad

Preparation Time: 10 minutes

Cooking Time: 15 minutes

Servings: 8

Ingredients:

- 1 c. orzo pasta, uncooked

- ½ c. freshly minced parsley

- 6 tsp. divided olive oil

- 1 onion, finely chopped

- 1½ tsp. Oregano, dried

- 1/3 c. red wine vinegar

- Salt

Directions:

1. Cook and drain the orzo. Add it to a serving dish with two teaspoons of the oil.

2. In another dish mix the parsley, onion, salt, vinegar, sugar, rest of the oil, oregano, and pepper. Pour over the orzo and place it in the fridge for two to 24 hours.

3. Right before the time for lunch, blend in the olives, tomatoes, cucumber, and cheese. Serve with a smile!

Nutrition:

399 calories

12.7g fat

55g carbs

16.2g protein

35. Mediterranean Egg Salad

Preparation Time: 10 minutes

Cooking Time: 8 minutes

Servings: 4

Ingredients:

- 8 eggs, hard-boiled

- ½ c. Chopped cucumber

- ½ c. Red onion

- ½ c. tomatoes, Sun-dried

- ¼ c. olives

- Splash – lemon juice

- ½ c. plain Greek yogurt

- ¼ tsp. cumin

- 1½ tsp. oregano

- Freshly cracked black pepper

- ½ tsp. sea salt

Directions:

1. Drain off the excess of oil from the tomatoes. Chop the veggies and eggs.

2. Combine the eggs with the tomatoes, onion, olives, and cucumber. Stir in the spices, lemon juice, and yogurt.

3. Refrigerate for about one week.

Nutrition:

240 calories

23g fat

3g carbs

7g protein

36. Mediterranean Pasta Salad

Preparation Time: 15 minutes

Cooking Time: 10 minutes

Servings: 4

Ingredients:

- 8 oz. multigrain farfalle

- 2 tsp. olive oil

- 1 lemon – Zest & juice

- 13.5 oz. artichoke hearts

- 8 oz. mozzarella cheese, freshly chopped

- ¼ c. chopped Red bell pepper, roasted

- ¼ c. freshly chopped parsley

- ½ c. frozen peas

Directions:

1. Prepare the pasta according to package directions (omit fat and salt).

2. Combine the zest, juiced lemon, and oil in a mixing container.

3. Drain and chop the artichoke. Add it and the rest of the fixings (cheese, parsley, and peppers). Toss well.

4. Add the peas to a colander. Pour the pasta and water over it when it's done. Shake to drain (don't run water over). Add to the mixture and toss.

5. Serve and enjoy at room temperature or warmed.

Nutrition:

159 calories

3.5g fat

26g carbs

5.7g protein

37. Mediterranean Quinoa Salad

Preparation Time: 10 minutes

Cooking Time: 15-20 minutes

Servings: 4

Ingredients:

- 1 c. uncooked quinoa

- 1/3 c. red wine vinegar

- 2 c. water

- ¼ c. olive oil

- 1 red pepper, diced

- 1 red onion, diced

- ½ c. Kalamata olives

- 1 juiced lemon

- ½ c. freshly chopped cilantro

- ½ tsp. black pepper

- 1 tsp. salt

- ½ c. crumbled feta cheese

- 2 Roma tomatoes

Directions:

1. First, you will need to dice the tomatoes, onions, and peppers.

2. Prepare a pot of water (med. heat) to boil, and add the quinoa. Reduce the heat and cook for 15-20 minutes. The water should be completely absorbed. Fluff and cool for five minutes.

3. Add the vinegar and oil—as the quinoa comes to room temperature.

4. Blend in the tomatoes, onion, olives, red peppers, cilantro, pepper, and salt. Gently blend and add the feta cheese. Refrigerate for about two hours so the flavors can intertwine.

5. Before serving, give it a drizzle of lemon juice.

Nutrition:

192 calories

7.6g fat

19.7g carbs

10.7g protein

38. Mexican Tuna Salad

Preparation Time: 10 minutes

Cooking Time: 5 minutes

Servings: 2

Ingredients:

- 6 oz. chunk light tuna in water

- 2 scallions, minced

- 1 green pepper, minced

- ¼ c. prepared green salsa

- 6 chopped pimento olives, stuffed

- 1 tbsp. lime juice

- 2 tbsps. mayonnaise, reduced-fat

- ½ tsp. ground cumin

- Ground black pepper

Directions:

1. Combine all of the fixings in a dish. Season with the pepper and salt.

2. Enjoy however you like it!

Nutrition:

188 calories

9.6g fat

19.7g carbs

10.5g protein

39. Spinach & Tuna Salad

Preparation Time: 10 minutes

Cooking Time: 5 minutes

Servings: 1

Ingredients:

- 1½ tbsps. Water

- 1½ tbsps. Lemon juice

- 1½ tbsps. Tahini

- 5 oz. chunk light tuna

- 4 Kalamata olives pitted

- 2 tbsps. Parsley

- 2 tbsps. Feta cheese

- 2 c. baby spinach

- 1 orange

Directions:

1. Drain the tuna and chop the olives. Whisk the water, juice, and tahini together. Blend in the rest of the fixings – stirring well to combine.

2. Serve over the baby spinach with the orange peeled and sliced on the side.

Nutrition:

203 calories

9g fat

14.7g carbs

9.5g protein

40. Tuscan Style Tuna Salad

Preparation Time: 10 minutes

Cooking Time: 5 minutes

Servings: 4

Ingredients:

- 15 oz. small white beans

- 6 oz. drained chunk light tuna

- 10 cherry tomatoes, quartered

- 4 trimmed scallions, sliced

- ¼ tsp. salt

- 2 tbsps. lemon juice

- Pepper

Directions:

1. Combine all of the fixings in a covered container.

2. Stir gently and refrigerate until ready to eat.

Nutrition:

322 calories

8.2g fat

32.9g carbs

30g protein

41. Chicken Souvlaki With Tzatziki

Preparation Time: 10 minutes

Cooking Time: 10-12 minutes

Servings: 6

Ingredients:

- 2 tbsps. lemon juice

- 14 oz. Greek yogurt

- 2 tsp. chopped oregano leaves

- ¼ c. white dry wine

- ¼ c. olive oil

- ½ tsp. pepper - divided

- 1 tsp. kosher salt

- 2 lb. skinned breasts

- 4 minced garlic cloves

- 2 tsp. distilled white vinegar

- ½ c. cucumber

Directions:

1. Cut the chicken into ½-inch cubes, and coarsely shred

the cucumber.

2. Set the grill between 450ºF and 550ºF.

3. Blend the wine, oil, chicken, oregano, lemon juice, cloves, ¼ teaspoon of the pepper, and the salt in a mixing bowl.

4. Use eight metal skewers to prepare the chicken for cooking. Grill for approximately 10-12 minutes.

5. Remove any excess moisture from the cucumbers with paper towels, and put them into a medium dish. Mix in the yogurt, garlic, vinegar, and pepper with the cucumbers.

6. Serve with warm pita bread and the chicken.

Nutrition:

294 calories

5.2g fat

42.1g carbs

22.2g protein

42. Creamy Paninis

Preparation Time: 10 minutes

Cooking Time: 5 minutes

Servings: 4

Ingredients:

- 8 slices whole-grain bread

- ½ c. mayonnaise

- ¼ c. fresh basil leaves

- 7-oz. roasted red peppers

- 2 tbsps. chopped black olives

- 1 sliced zucchini

- 4 slices provolone cheese

Directions:

1. Finely chop the basil leaves.

2. In a small dish, mix the finely chopped olives with the mayonnaise.

3. Spread it on the slices of bread with the peppers, zucchini, and provolone. Top with the remainder of the slices.

4. Place mayonnaise on the outside of each sandwich.

5. On the stovetop using medium heat, place the sandwiches on a grill pan or skillet. Brown each of the sandwiches for approximately four minutes.

6. What a treat with all of that melted cheese!

Nutrition:

300 calories

44g fat

33g carbs

26g protein

43. Pressed Picnic Sandwich

Preparation Time: 15 minutes

Cooking Time: 10 minutes

Servings: 6

Ingredients:

- 1 small zucchini

- 1 small eggplant

- 1 small yellow squash

- 3 tbsp. olive oil

- 1 large ciabatta bread

- 1/3 c. tapenade

- 1/3 c. pesto

- 2 jars sliced and roasted red peppers

- 18 oz. mozzarella

- 2 tbsp. balsamic vinegar

Directions:

1. Slice the veggies lengthwise into ¼- inch slices. Drain and slice the mozzarella. Warm up the grill or grill pan (med.-high).

2. Use a brush to lightly oil the veggies. Grill 3-4 minutes for each side, until softened and charred. Arrange on a platter.

3. Prepare the bread with pesto on one side and the tapenade on the other.

4. Layer the veggies and mozzarella on one side and drizzle with the rest of the oil and vinegar. Shake the pepper and salt as desired.

5. Press the sandwich together and wrap tightly using plastic wrap. Refrigerate on a baking tin overnight or at least two hours. Apply a heavy skillet to 'squash' the sandwich.

6. When ready to serve, unwrap and slice.

Nutrition:

766 calories

31g fat

60g carbs

44. Roasted Peppers With Broiled Feta & Olives

Preparation Time: 15 minutes

Cooking Time: 20minutes

Servings: 6

Ingredients:

- 1 yellow

- 1 red pepper

- 1 Vidalia onion

- 1 tsp. olive oil

- 1 head garlic

- 1 tbsp. regular capers or 8 caper berries

- 12 green olives

- 8 anchovies

- 12 Kalamata olives

- Juice of 1 lemon

- 8 oz. feta cheese

- ¼ c. chives

- ¼ c. mint

- ¼ c. dill

- ¼ c.

Directions:

1. Slice the peppers into halves, lengthwise. Separate the cloves and peel. Slice the onion into rounds. Warm up the oven to 400ºF.

2. Arrange the garlic, onion, and peppers on a baking sheet. Brush them with some oil and bake (approximately 20 min.). Take from the oven, place on a covered dish or under some tight-fitting wrap.

3. Reset the broiler setting in the oven. Use a baking sheet or casserole dish to crumble the feta. Broil until it bubbles - approximately two minutes.

4. Blend the remaining ingredients in a large mixing dish. Combine the onions, garlic, and peppers - tossing well.

5. Take the cheese from the broiler and spoon into the serving plates. Garnish with the pepper mixture.

Nutrition:

221 calories

20g fat

4g carbs

8g protein

45. Spinach With Garbanzo Beans

Preparation Time: 10 minutes

Cooking Time: 5 minutes

Servings: 4

Ingredients:

- 1 tbsp. olive oil

- 4 minced garlic cloves

- ½ diced onion

- 10 oz. chopped spinach

- 12 oz. garbanzo beans

- ½ tsp. cumin

- ½ tsp. salt

Directions:

1. In a skillet, warm the olive oil over medium-low heat.

2. Then add the onions, and garlic and cook until the onions are translucent. About 5 minutes.

3. Stir in spinach, cumin, salt, and garbanzo beans. Use your

spoon to slightly mash the beans as the mixture cooks.

4. Allow cooking until thoroughly heated.

Nutrition:

90 calories

4g fat

11g carbs

4g protein

46. Grilled Oregano Chicken Kebabs With Zucchini And Olives

Preparation Time: 10 minutes

Cooking Time: 20 minutes

Servings: 4

Ingredients:

- Nonstick cooking spray

- ¼ cup extra-virgin olive oil

- 2 tablespoons balsamic vinegar

- 1 teaspoon dried oregano, crushed between your fingers

- 1 pound boneless, skinless chicken breasts, cut into 1½-inch pieces

- 2 medium zucchini, cut into 1-inch pieces (about 2½ cups)

- ½ cup Kalamata olives pitted and halved

- 2 tablespoons olive brine

- ¼ cup torn fresh basil leaves

Directions:

1. Coat the cold grill with nonstick cooking spray. Heat the grill to medium-high.

2. In a small bowl, whisk together the oil, vinegar, and oregano. Divide the marinade between two large plastic zip-top bags.

3. Add the chicken to one bag and the zucchini to another. Seal and massage the marinade into both the chicken and zucchini.

4. Thread the chicken onto 6 (12-inch) wooden skewers. Thread the zucchini onto 8 or 9 (12-inch) wooden skewers. Cook the kebabs in batches on the grill for 5 minutes, flip, and grill for 5 minutes more, until any chicken juices, run clear.

5. Remove the chicken and zucchini from the skewers and put them in a large serving bowl. Toss with the olives,

olive brine, and basil and serve.

Nutrition:

Calories: 264

Total Fat: 16g

Saturated Fat: 2g

Cholesterol: 65mg

Sodium: 209mg

Total Carbohydrates: 5g

Fiber: 2g

Protein: 27g

47. Honey Almond–Crusted Chicken Tenders

Preparation Time: 10 minutes

Cooking Time: 20 minutes

Servings: 4

Ingredients:

- Nonstick cooking spray

- 1 tablespoon honey

- 1 tablespoon whole-grain or Dijon mustard

- ¼ teaspoon kosher or sea salt

- ¼ teaspoon freshly ground black pepper

- 1 pound boneless, skinless chicken breast tenders or tenderloins

- 1 cup almonds (about 3 ounces)

Directions:

1. Preheat the oven to 425°F. Line a large, rimmed baking sheet with parchment paper. Place a wire cooling rack on the parchment-lined baking sheet, and coat the rack well with nonstick cooking spray.

2. In a large bowl, combine the honey, mustard, salt, and

pepper. Add the chicken and stir gently to coat. Set aside.

3. Use a knife or a mini food processor to roughly chop the almonds; they should be about the size of sunflower seeds. Dump the nuts onto a large sheet of parchment paper and spread them out. Press the coated chicken tenders into the nuts until evenly coated on all sides. Place the chicken on the prepared wire rack.

4. Bake for 15 to 20 minutes, or until the internal temperature of the chicken measures 165°F on a meat thermometer and any juices run clear. Serve immediately.

Nutrition:

Calories: 263

Total Fat: 12g

Saturated Fat: 1g

Cholesterol: 65mg

Sodium: 237mg

Total Carbohydrates: 9g

Fiber: 3g

Protein: 31g

48. One-Pan Parsley Chicken And Potatoes

Preparation Time: 10 minutes

Cooking Time: 25 minutes

Servings: 6

Ingredients:

- 1½ pounds boneless, skinless chicken thighs, cut into 1-inch cubes

- 1 tablespoon extra-virgin olive oil

- 1½ pounds Yukon Gold potatoes, unpeeled, cut into ½-inch cubes (about 6 small potatoes)

- 2 garlic cloves, minced (about 1 teaspoon)

- ¼ cup dry white wine or apple cider vinegar

- 1 cup low-sodium or no-salt-added chicken broth

- 1 tablespoon Dijon mustard

- ¼ teaspoon kosher or sea salt

- ¼ teaspoon freshly ground black pepper

- 1 cup chopped fresh flat-leaf (Italian) parsley, including stems

- 1 tablespoon freshly squeezed lemon juice (½ small lemon)

Directions:

1. Pat the chicken dry with a few paper towels. In a large skillet over medium-high heat, heat the oil. Add the chicken and cook for 5 minutes, stirring only after the chicken has browned on one side. Remove the chicken from the pan with a slotted spoon, and put it on a plate; it will not yet be fully cooked. Leave the skillet on the stove.

2. Add the potatoes to the skillet and cook for 5 minutes, stirring only after the potatoes have become golden and crispy on one side. Push the potatoes to the side of the skillet, add the garlic, and cook, stirring constantly, for 1

minute. Add the wine and cook for 1 minute, until nearly evaporated. Add the chicken broth, mustard, salt, pepper, and reserved chicken pieces. Turn the heat up to high, and bring to a boil.

3. Once boiling, cover the skillet, reduce the heat to medium-low, and cook for 10 to 12 minutes, until the potatoes are tender and the internal temperature of the chicken measures 165°F on a meat thermometer and any juices run clear.

4. During the last minute of cooking, stir in the parsley. Remove from the heat, stir in the lemon juice, and serve.

Nutrition:

Calories: 241

Total Fat: 4g

Saturated Fat: 1g

Cholesterol: 65mg

Sodium: 245mg

Total Carbohydrates: 20g

Fiber: 3g

Protein: 29g

49. Romesco Poached Chicken

Preparation Time: 10 minutes

Cooking Time: 20 minutes

Servings: 6

Ingredients:

- 1½ pounds boneless, skinless chicken breasts, cut into 6 pieces

- 1 carrot, halved

- 1 celery stalk, halved

- ½ onion halved

- 2 garlic cloves, smashed

- 3 sprigs fresh thyme or rosemary

- 1 cup Romesco Dip

- 2 tablespoons chopped fresh flat-leaf (Italian) parsley

- ¼ teaspoon freshly ground black pepper

Directions:

1. Put the chicken in a medium saucepan. Fill with water until there's about one inch of liquid above the chicken. Add the carrot, celery, onion, garlic, and thyme. Cover

and bring it to a boil. Reduce the heat to low (keeping it covered), and cook for 12 to 15 minutes, or until the internal temperature of the chicken measures 165°F on a meat thermometer and any juices run clear.

2. Remove the chicken from the water and let sit for 5 minutes.

3. When you're ready to serve, spread ¾ cup of romesco dip on the bottom of a serving platter. Arrange the chicken breasts on top, and drizzle with the remaining romesco dip. Sprinkle the tops with parsley and pepper.

Nutrition:

Calories: 237

Total Fat: 11g

Saturated Fat: 1g

Cholesterol: 65mg

Sodium: 336mg

Total Carbohydrates: 8g

Fiber: 4g

Protein: 28g

50. Roasted Red Pepper Chicken With Lemony Garlic Hummus

Preparation Time: 10 minutes

Cooking Time: 10 minutes

Servings: 6

Ingredients:

- 1¼ pounds boneless, skinless chicken thighs, cut into 1-inch pieces

- ½ sweet or red onion, cut into 1-inch chunks (about 1 cup)

- 2 tablespoons extra-virgin olive oil

- ½ teaspoon dried thyme

- ¼ teaspoon freshly ground black pepper

- ¼ teaspoon kosher or sea salt

- 1 (12-ounce) jar roasted red peppers, drained and chopped

- Lemony Garlic Hummus, or a 10-ounce container prepared hummus

- ½ medium lemon

- 3 (6-inch) whole-wheat pita bread, cut into eighths

Directions:

1. Line a large, rimmed baking sheet with aluminum foil. Set aside. Set one oven rack about 4 inches below the broiler element. Preheat the broiler to high.

2. In a large bowl, mix the chicken, onion, oil, thyme, pepper, and salt. Spread the mixture onto the prepared baking sheet.

3. Place the chicken under the broiler and broil for 5 minutes. Remove the pan, stir in the red peppers, and return to the broiler. Broil for another 5 minutes, or until the chicken and onion just start to char on the tips. Remove from the oven.

4. Spread the hummus onto a large serving platter, and spoon the chicken mixture on top. Squeeze the juice from half a lemon over the top, and serve with the pita pieces.

Nutrition:

Calories: 324

Total Fat: 11g

Saturated Fat: 2g

Cholesterol: 54mg

Sodium: 625mg

Total Carbohydrates: 29g

Fiber: 6g

Protein: 29g

51. Moroccan Meatballs

Preparation Time: 10 minutes

Cooking Time: 20 minutes

Servings: 4

Ingredients:

- ¼ cup finely chopped onion (about ⅛ onion)

- ¼ cup raisins, coarsely chopped

- 1 teaspoon ground cumin

- ½ teaspoon ground cinnamon

- ¼ teaspoon smoked paprika

- 1 large egg

- 1 pound ground beef (93% lean) or ground lamb

- ⅓ cup panko bread crumbs

- 1 teaspoon extra-virgin olive oil

- 1 (28-ounce) can low-sodium or no-salt-added crushed tomatoes

- Chopped fresh mint, feta cheese, and/or fresh orange or lemon wedges, for serving (optional)

Directions:

1. In a large bowl, combine the onion, raisins, cumin, cinnamon, smoked paprika, and egg. Add the ground beef and bread crumbs and mix gently with your hands. Divide the mixture into 20 even portions, then wet your hands and roll each portion into a ball. Wash your hands.

2. In a large skillet over medium-high heat, heat the oil. Add the meatballs and cook for 8 minutes, rolling around every minute or so with tongs or a fork to brown them on most sides. (They won't be cooked through.) Transfer the meatballs to a paper towel-lined plate. Drain the fat out of the pan, and carefully wipe out the hot pan with a paper towel.

3. Return the meatballs to the pan, and pour the tomatoes over the meatballs. Cover and cook on medium-high heat until the sauce begins to bubble. Lower the heat to medium, cover partially, and cook for 7 to 8 more minutes, until the meatballs are cooked through. Garnish with fresh mint, feta cheese, and/or a squeeze of citrus, if desired, and serve.

Nutrition:

Calories: 306

Total Fat: 10g

Saturated Fat: 4g

Cholesterol: 117mg

Sodium: 342mg

Total Carbohydrates: 26g

Fiber: 7g

Protein: 29g

52. Beef Spanakopita Pita Pockets

Preparation Time: 5 minutes

Cooking Time: 15 minutes

Servings: 4

Ingredients:

- 3 teaspoons extra-virgin olive oil, divided

- 1 pound ground beef (93% lean)

- 2 garlic cloves, minced (about 1 teaspoon)

- 2 (6-ounce) bags baby spinach, chopped (about 12 cups)

- ½ cup crumbled feta cheese (about 2 ounces)

- ⅓ cup ricotta cheese

- ½ teaspoon ground nutmeg

- ¼ teaspoon freshly ground black pepper

- ¼ cup slivered almonds

- 4 (6-inch) whole-wheat pita bread, cut in half

Directions:

1. In a large skillet over medium heat, heat 1 teaspoon of oil. Add the ground beef and cook for 10 minutes, breaking it up with a wooden spoon and stirring occasionally. Remove from the heat and drain in a colander. Set the meat aside.

2. Place the skillet back on the heat, and add the remaining 2 teaspoons of oil. Add the garlic and cook for 1 minute, stirring constantly. Add the spinach and cook for 2 to 3 minutes, or until the spinach has cooked down, stirring often.

3. Turn off the heat and mix in the feta cheese, ricotta, nutmeg, and pepper. Stir until all the ingredients are well incorporated. Mix in the almonds.

4. Divide the beef filling among the eight pita pocket halves to stuff them and serve.

Nutrition:

Calories: 506
Total Fat: 22g

Saturated Fat: 8g

Cholesterol: 98mg

Sodium: 567mg

Total Carbohydrates: 42g

Fiber: 8g

Protein: 39g

53. Grilled Steak, Mushroom, And Onion Kebabs

Preparation Time: 10 minutes

Cooking Time: 10 minutes

Servings: 4

Ingredients:

- Nonstick cooking spray

- 4 garlic cloves, peeled

- 2 fresh rosemary sprigs (about 3 inches each)

- 2 tablespoons extra-virgin olive oil, divided

- 1 pound boneless top sirloin steak, about 1 inch thick

- 1 (8-ounce) package white button mushrooms

- 1 medium red onion, cut into 12 thin wedges

- ¼ teaspoon coarsely ground black pepper

- 2 tablespoons red wine vinegar

- ¼ teaspoon kosher or sea salt

Directions:

1. Soak 12 (10-inch) wooden skewers in water. Spray the cold grill with nonstick cooking spray, and heat the grill

to medium-high.

2. Cut a piece of aluminum foil into a 10-inch square. Place the garlic and rosemary sprigs in the center, drizzle with 1 tablespoon of oil, and wrap tightly to form a foil packet. Place it on the grill, and close the grill cover.

3. Cut the steak into 1-inch cubes. Thread the beef onto the wet skewers, alternating with whole mushrooms and onion wedges. Spray the kebabs thoroughly with nonstick cooking spray, and sprinkle with pepper.

4. Cook the kebabs on the covered grill for 4 to 5 minutes. Turn and grill 4 to 5 more minutes, covered, until a meat thermometer inserted in the meat registers 145°F (medium-rare) or 160°F (medium).

5. Remove the foil packet from the grill, open, and, using tongs, place the garlic and rosemary sprigs in a small bowl. Carefully strip the rosemary sprigs of their leaves into the bowl and pour in any accumulated juices and oil from the foil packet. Add the remaining 1 tablespoon of oil and the vinegar and salt. Mash the garlic with a fork, and mix all ingredients in the bowl together. Pour over the finished steak kebabs and serve.

Nutrition:

Calories: 300

Total Fat: 14g

Saturated Fat: 4g

Cholesterol: 101mg

Sodium: 196mg

Total Carbohydrates: 6g

Fiber: 1g

Protein: 36g

54. Beef Gyros With Tahini Sauce

Preparation Time: 15 minutes

Cooking Time: 10 minutes

Servings: 4

Ingredients:

- Nonstick cooking spray

- 2 tablespoons extra-virgin olive oil

- 1 tablespoon dried oregano

- 1¼ teaspoons garlic powder, divided

- 1 teaspoon ground cumin

- ½ teaspoon freshly ground black pepper

- ¼ teaspoon kosher or sea salt

- 1 pound beef flank steak, top round steak, or lamb leg steak, center cut, about 1 inch thick

- 1 medium green bell pepper, halved and seeded

- 2 tablespoons tahini or peanut butter (tahini for nut-free)

- 1 tablespoon hot water (if needed)

- ½ cup 2% plain Greek yogurt

- 1 tablespoon freshly squeezed lemon juice (about ½ small lemon)

- 1 cup thinly sliced red onion (about ½ onion)

- 4 (6-inch) whole-wheat pita bread, warmed

Directions:

1. Set an oven rack about 4 inches below the broiler element. Preheat the oven broiler to high. Line a large, rimmed baking sheet with foil. Place a wire cooling rack on the foil, and spray the rack with nonstick cooking spray. Set aside.

2. In a small bowl, whisk together the oil, oregano, 1 teaspoon of garlic powder, cumin, pepper, and salt. Rub the oil mixture on all sides of the steak, saving 1

teaspoon of the mixture. Place the steak on the prepared rack. Rub the remaining oil mixture on the bell pepper, and place on the rack, cut-side down. Press the pepper with the heel of your hand to flatten.

3. Broil for 5 minutes. Turn the meat and the pepper pieces, and broil for 2 to 5 more minutes, until the pepper is charred and the internal temperature of the meat measures 145°F on a meat thermometer. Put the pepper and steak on a cutting board to rest for 5 minutes.

4. While the meat is broiling, in a small bowl, whisk the tahini until smooth (adding 1 tablespoon of hot water if your tahini is sticky). Add the remaining ¼ teaspoon of garlic powder and the yogurt and lemon juice, and whisk thoroughly.

5. Slice the steak crosswise into ¼-inch-thick strips. Slice the bell pepper into strips. Divide the steak, bell pepper, and onion among the warm pita bread. Drizzle with tahini sauce and serve.

Nutrition:

Calories: 497

Total Fat: 21g

Saturated Fat: 5g

Cholesterol: 53mg

Sodium: 548mg

Total Carbohydrates: 45g

Fiber: 7g

Protein: 36g

55. Beef Sliders With Pepper Slaw

Preparation Time: 10 minutes

Cooking Time: 10 minutes

Servings: 4

Ingredients:

- Nonstick cooking spray

- 1 (8-ounce) package white button mushrooms

- 2 tablespoons extra-virgin olive oil, divided

- 1 pound ground beef (93% lean)

- 2 garlic cloves, minced (about 1 teaspoon)

- ½ teaspoon kosher or sea salt, divided

- ¼ teaspoon freshly ground black pepper

- 1 tablespoon balsamic vinegar

- 2 bell peppers of different colors, sliced into strips

- 2 tablespoons torn fresh basil or flat-leaf (Italian) parsley

- Mini or slider whole-grain rolls, for serving (optional)

Directions:

1. Set one oven rack about 4 inches below the broiler element. Preheat the oven broiler to high.

2. Line a large, rimmed baking sheet with aluminum foil. Place a wire cooling rack on the aluminum foil, and spray the rack with nonstick cooking spray. Set aside.

3. Put half the mushrooms in the bowl of a food processor and pulse about 15 times, until the mushrooms are finely chopped but not puréed, similar to the texture of ground meat. Repeat with the remaining mushrooms.

4. In a large skillet over medium-high heat, heat 1 tablespoon of oil. Add the mushrooms and cook for 2 to 3 minutes, stirring occasionally, until the mushrooms have cooked down and some of their liquid has evaporated. Remove from the heat.

5. In a large bowl, combine the ground beef with the cooked mushrooms, garlic, ¼ teaspoon of salt, and pepper. Mix gently using your hands. Form the meat into 8 small (½-inch-thick) patties, and place on the

prepared rack, making two lines of 4 patties down the center of the pan.

6. Place the pan in the oven so the broiler heating element is directly over as many burgers as possible. Broil for 4 minutes. Flip the burgers and rearrange them so any burgers not getting brown are nearer to the heat source. Broil for 3 to 4 more minutes, or until the internal temperature of the meat is 160°F on a meat thermometer. Watch carefully to prevent burning.

7. While the burgers are cooking, in a large bowl, whisk together the remaining 1 tablespoon of oil, vinegar, and remaining ¼ teaspoon of salt. Add the peppers and basil, and stir gently to coat with the dressing. Serve the sliders with the pepper slaw as a topping or on the side. If desired, serve with the rolls, burger style.

Nutrition:

Calories: 259

Total Fat: 15g

Saturated Fat: 4g

Cholesterol: 73mg

Sodium: 315mg

Total Carbohydrates: 5g

Fiber: 2g

Protein: 26g

56. Shrimp Scampi

Preparation Time: 10 minutes

Cooking Time: 15 minutes

Servings: 4

Ingredients:

- 2 tablespoons extra-virgin olive oil

- 1 shallot, minced

- 1 pound medium shrimp, peeled, deveined, and tails removed

- 6 garlic cloves, minced

- Juice of 1 lemon

- Zest of 1 lemon

- ½ cup dry white wine

- ½ teaspoon of sea salt

- ¼ teaspoon freshly ground black pepper

- Pinch red pepper flakes

- ¼ cup chopped fresh Italian parsley leaves

- 6 ounces whole-wheat pasta, cooked according to package directions

Directions:

1. In a large skillet over medium-high heat, heat the olive oil until it shimmers.

2. Add the shallot. Cook for about 5 minutes, stirring occasionally, until soft.

3. Toss in the shrimp. Cook for 3 to 4 minutes, stirring occasionally until the shrimp is pink.

4. Add the garlic and cook for 30 seconds, stirring constantly.

5. Stir in the lemon juice and zest, wine, sea salt, pepper, and red pepper flakes. Bring to a simmer and reduce the heat to medium-low. Cook for about 2 minutes until the liquid reduces by half. Remove from the heat and stir in the parsley.

6. Toss with the hot pasta and serve.

Nutrition:

Calories: 394

Protein: 32g

Total Carbohydrates: 38g

Sugars: 2g

Fiber: 4g

Total Fat: 10g

Saturated Fat: 2g

Cholesterol: 239mg

Sodium: 524mg

57. Shrimp Mojo De Ajo

Preparation Time: 10 minutes

Cooking Time: 40 minutes

Servings: 4

Ingredients:

- ¼ cup extra-virgin olive oil

- 10 garlic cloves, minced

- ⅛ teaspoon cayenne pepper, plus more as needed

- 8 ounces mushrooms, quartered

- 1 pound medium shrimp, peeled, deveined, and tails removed

- Juice of 1 lime

- ½ teaspoon of sea salt

- ¼ cup chopped fresh cilantro leaves

- 2 cups cooked brown rice

Directions:

1. In a small saucepan over the lowest heat setting, bring the olive oil, garlic, and cayenne to a low simmer so bubbles just barely break the surface of the oil. Simmer

for 30 minutes, stirring occasionally. Strain the garlic from the oil and set it aside.

2. Add the olive oil to a large skillet over medium-high heat and heat it until it shimmers.

3. Add the mushrooms. Cook for about 5 minutes, stirring once or twice until browned.

4. Add the shrimp, lime juice, and sea salt. Cook for about 4 minutes, stirring occasionally until the shrimp are pink.

5. Remove from the heat and stir in the cilantro and reserved garlic. Serve over the hot brown rice.

Nutrition:

Calories: 354

Protein: 30g

Total Carbohydrates: 24g

Sugars: 1g

Fiber: 2g

Total Fat: 15g

Saturated Fat: 3g

Cholesterol: 239mg

Sodium: 518mg

58. Pan-Seared Scallops With Sautéed Spinach

Preparation Time: 15 minutes

Cooking Time: 10 minutes

Servings: 4

Ingredients:

- 1 pound sea scallops (see tip)

- 1 teaspoon sea salt, divided

- ½ teaspoon freshly ground black pepper, divided

- 2 tablespoons extra-virgin olive oil

- 6 cups fresh baby spinach

- Juice of 1 orange

- Pinch red pepper flakes

Directions:

1. Season the scallops on both sides with ½ teaspoon of sea salt and ¼ teaspoon of pepper.

2. In a large skillet over medium-high heat, heat the olive oil until it shimmers.

3. Add the scallops. Cook for 3 to 4 minutes per side without moving until browned. Remove the scallops

from the skillet and set aside, tented with aluminum foil to keep warm.

4. Return the skillet to the heat and add the spinach, orange juice, red pepper flakes, remaining ½ teaspoon of salt, and remaining ¼ teaspoon of pepper. Cook for 4 to 5 minutes, stirring, until the spinach wilts.

5. Divide the spinach among 4 plates and top with the scallops. Serve immediately.

Nutrition:

Calories: 186

Protein: 21g

Total Carbohydrates: 8g

Sugars: 3g

Fiber: 2g

Total Fat: 8g

Saturated Fat: <1g

Cholesterol: 37mg

Sodium: 686mg

59. Pasta Puttanesca

Preparation Time: 10 minutes

Cooking Time: 10 minutes

Servings: 4

Ingredients:

- 2 tablespoons extra-virgin olive oil

- 6 garlic cloves, finely minced (or put through a garlic press)

- 2 teaspoons anchovy paste

- ¼ teaspoon red pepper flakes, plus more as needed

- 20 black olives, pitted and chopped

- 3 tablespoons capers, drained and rinsed

- ¼ teaspoon of sea salt

- ¼ teaspoon freshly ground black pepper

- 2 (14-ounce) cans crushed tomatoes, undrained

- 1 (14-ounce) can chopped tomatoes, drained

- ¼ cup chopped fresh basil leaves

- 8 ounces whole-wheat spaghetti, cooked according to

package instructions and drained

Directions:

1. In a sauté pan or skillet over medium heat, stir together the olive oil, garlic, anchovy paste, and red pepper flakes. Cook for about 2 minutes, stirring, until the mixture is very fragrant.

2. Add the olives, capers, sea salt, and pepper.

3. In a blender, purée the crushed and chopped tomatoes and add to the pan. Cook for about 5 minutes, stirring occasionally until the mixture simmers.

4. Stir in the basil and cooked pasta. Toss to coat the pasta with the sauce and serve.

Nutrition:

Calories: 278

Protein: 10g

Total Carbohydrates: 40g

Sugars: 16g

Fiber: 12g

Total Fat: 13g

Saturated Fat: 1g

Cholesterol: 9mg

Sodium: 1,099mg

60. Pasta With Pesto

- Preparation Time: 10 minutes

- Cooking Time: 0 minutes

- Servings: 4

- Ingredients:

- 3 tablespoons extra-virgin olive oil

- 3 garlic cloves, finely minced

- ½ cup fresh basil leaves

- ¼ cup (about 2 ounces) grated Parmesan cheese

- ¼ cup pine nuts

- 8 ounces whole-wheat pasta, cooked according to package instructions and drained

Directions:

1. In a blender or food processor, combine the olive oil, garlic, basil, cheese, and pine nuts. Pulse for 10 to 20 (1-second) pulses until everything is chopped and blended.

2. Toss with the hot pasta and serve.

Nutrition:

Calories: 405

Protein: 13g

Total Carbohydrates: 44g

Sugars: 2g

Fiber: 5g

Total Fat: 21g

Saturated Fat: 4g

Cholesterol: 10mg

Sodium: 141mg

61. Greek Meatballs (Keftedes)

Preparation Time: 20 minutes

Cooking Time: 25 minutes

Servings: 4

Ingredients:

- 2 whole-wheat bread slices

- 1¼ pounds ground turkey

- 1 egg

- ¼ cup seasoned whole-wheat bread crumbs

- 3 garlic cloves, minced

- ¼ red onion, grated

- ¼ cup chopped fresh Italian parsley leaves

- 2 tablespoons chopped fresh mint leaves

- 2 tablespoons chopped fresh oregano leaves

- ½ teaspoon of sea salt

- ¼ teaspoon freshly ground black pepper

Directions:

1. Preheat the oven to 350°F.

2. Line a baking sheet with parchment paper or aluminum foil.

3. Run the bread underwater to wet it, and squeeze out any excess. Tear the wet bread into small pieces and place it in a medium bowl.

4. Add the turkey, egg, bread crumbs, garlic, red onion, parsley, mint, oregano, sea salt, and pepper. Mix well. Form the mixture into ¼-cup-size balls. Place the meatballs on the prepared sheet and bake for about 25 minutes, or until the internal temperature reaches 165°F.

Nutrition:

Calories: 350

Protein: 42g

Total Carbohydrates: 10g

Sugars: 1g

Fiber: 3g

Total Fat: 18g

Saturated Fat: 3g

Cholesterol: 186mg

Sodium: 493mg

62. Lamb With String Beans (Arni Me Fasolakia)

Preparation Time: 10 minutes

Cooking Time: 1 hour

Servings: 6

Ingredients:

- ¼ cup extra-virgin olive oil, divided

- 6 lamb chops, trimmed of extra fat

- 1 teaspoon sea salt, divided

- ½ teaspoon freshly ground black pepper

- 2 tablespoons tomato paste

- 1½ cups hot water

- 1 pound green beans, trimmed and halved crosswise

- 1 onion, chopped

- 2 tomatoes, chopped

Directions:

1. In a large skillet over medium-high heat, heat 2 tablespoons of olive oil until it shimmers.

2. Season the lamb chops with ½ teaspoon of sea salt and

⅛ teaspoon of pepper. Cook the lamb in the hot oil for about 4 minutes per side until browned on both sides. Transfer the meat to a platter and set aside.

3. Return the skillet to the heat and add the remaining 2 tablespoons of olive oil. Heat until it shimmers.

4. In a bowl, dissolve the tomato paste in the hot water. Add it to the hot skillet along with the green beans, onion, tomatoes, and the remaining ½ teaspoon of sea salt and ¼ teaspoon of pepper. Bring to a simmer, using the side of a spoon to scrape and fold in any browned bits from the bottom of the pan.

5. Return the lamb chops to the pan. Bring to a boil and reduce the heat to medium-low. Simmer for 45 minutes until the beans are soft, adding additional water as needed to adjust the thickness of the sauce.

Nutrition:

Calories: 439

Protein: 50g

Total Carbohydrates: 10g

Sugars: 4g

Fiber: 4g

Total Fat: 22g

Saturated Fat: 6g

Cholesterol: 153mg and Sodium: 456mg

CPSIA information can be obtained
at www.ICGtesting.com
Printed in the USA
BVHW041013150321
602551BV00006B/480